THREE BRAINS

How the Heart, Brain, and Gut
Influence Mental Health and Identity

KAREN JENSEN, ND

With foreword by Patrick Holford,
author of *Optimum Nutrition for the Mind*

Three Brains

How the Heart, Brain, and Gut Influence Mental Health and Identity

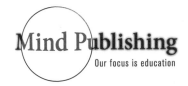

Mind Publishing
Our focus is education

FOR INFORMATION CONTACT:

Mind Publishing Inc.
PO Box 57559,
1031 Brunette Avenue
Coquitlam, BC Canada V3K 1E0
Tel: 604-777-4330 Toll free: 1-877-477-4904
Fax: 1-866-367-5508
Email: info@mindpublishing.com
mindpublishing.com

ISBN: 978-1-927017-22-7
Printed in Canada

Design: FWH Creative
Editor: Janice Dyer

This publication contains the ideas and opinions of its author. It is intended to provide helpful and informative material on the subjects addressed in the publication. It is sold with the understanding that the authors and the publisher are not engaged in rendering medical, health, or any other kind of personal professional services in the book. The reader should consult his or her medical, health, or other competent professional before adopting any of the suggestions in this book or drawing inferences from it.

The author and publisher specifically disclaim all responsibility for any liability, loss, or risk, personal or otherwise, which is incurred as a consequence, directly or indirectly, of the use and application of any of the contents of this book.

Table of Contents

Foreword

Two fundamentals for the developing brain are basic nutrition and a good education. You learn many things at school, but you never learn how your brain works, or how we actually have three brains that all work together to influence mental health and optimal wellness. All three brains are dependent on optimal nutrition. This book sets that error straight. By showing you how nutrients optimize your brain's function, Karen Jensen, a highly respected naturopathic doctor with years of experience helping people regain mental and physical health, gives you the essential keys for optimizing your experience of life.

One in four people experience a mental health problem at some point, from depression and memory loss to anxiety and insomnia. Even more experience feeling stressed. While issues in life are often a major driver of stress levels and mood swings, few people, including doctors, realize how suboptimal nutrition makes people less resilient and less able to cope with life's unavoidable challenges. As a consequence, they tend to overreact and get stuck in negative emotions and thought patterns. Also, they discover and use short-term fixes – stimulants such as caffeine and relaxants such as alcohol and other drugs – or are prescribed medications that, at best, fail to address the true underlying causes and, at worst, get them hooked and dependent, unable to quit without experiencing horrendous withdrawal effects.

Taking the time to learn how to optimize your three-brain function with the right diet and nutrients as well as simple but important lifestyle essentials, and knowing how to use supplements and herbs to restore mental well-being when you do go out of balance, is a "life essential" for anyone wanting a happy and healthy life and family. For more serious mental health problems, good psychotherapeutic guidance is also vital, yet few people realize that it too depends on healthy brain function.

Consider this book an essential read – as important as learning to cook or ride a bicycle. It is clearly laid out, comprehensive, and gives immediate solutions for a full range of mental health issues, so you will know what to do when you, a family member, or a friend hits troubled waters.

By following Dr. Jensen's advice you will have a faster, more energized brain, giving you clearer thought, more balanced emotions, better memory, better sleep, and increased resilience against stress and disease. There is no need for declining faculties with age. Alzheimer's, like diabetes, is a preventable disease, not an inevitable part of aging. Only 1% of all Alzheimer's cases are caused by genes. But unlike diabetes, it is not reversible. By following the advice in this book, you are investing in protecting your own mental health throughout life. That alone makes this book invaluable. In an enlightened world it should be essential reading for all.

Patrick Holford,

Founder of the Food for the Brain Foundation and the Institute for Optimum Nutrition, and author of *Optimum Nutrition for the Mind*.

Acknowledgments

Thank you to my three sons, who helped me to really know and understand the meaning of unconditional love.

Over the years my patients have been the fuel for the fire that has kept my passion alive in the field of medicine. It has been an honour to be part of their healing journey. By listening to them empathetically, I was able to keep in touch with both the art of medicine and the reality of medical practice – the patient experience versus the mountains of statistics. I also learned from them the reason for the terms "medical practice" and "patients": Patients need to have patience, while the doctors practice their skills in the art and science of medicine. Thank you for your patience over the years.

Finally, thank you to Roland Gahler, the owner of Natural Factors, for inviting me to be part of his vision.

Introduction

Brain-related conditions cross all levels of society. Although science has come a long way in understanding how the brain works, there is still much that we do not know. However, remarkable discoveries have been made over the past few decades about the brain's amazing ability to rewire itself, allowing the nerve cells to compensate and adapt to changes due to injury, disease, and other stressors. This area of discovery, called neuroplasticity, offers new opportunities and approaches to treating people with brain disorders. Also, thanks to an emerging science called epigenetics, researchers have learned that DNA no longer equals destiny – we each have the ability to influence how our genes express themselves. With healthy lifestyle choices, stress reduction, and nutritional supplementation, we can actually alter genetic expression. This is exciting news considering the ever-increasing number of people who are being diagnosed with mental health disorders and degenerative neurological diseases.

But, what if there were three brains all influencing each other to determine our state of mental emotional well-being and overall health? Research suggests that there are actually three brains: the heart brain, the gut brain, and the head brain.

The gut brain contains approximately 100 million neurons and it can work both independently of and in conjunction with the head brain. Even though there may not be conscious awareness that the gut is thinking, many people experience a "gut feeling" or "gut instinct". Studies indicate that the gut microbiota communicates with the head brain, affecting function and behaviour, and suggesting a role for the gut microbiota in the regulation of anxiety, mood, cognition, and pain. "A lot of the information that the gut sends to the brain affects well-being, and doesn't even come to consciousness", says Michael Gershon at Columbia-Presbyterian Medical Center, New York and author of *The Second Brain* (1998). Even though the gut-brain connection has been recognized in Western medicine since the mid-nineteenth century, the emerging field called neurogastroenterology, it is still new thinking for some.

The human heart, in addition to its other functions, actually possesses a heart-brain composed of about 40,000 neurons. Scientists initially became interested in the heart-brain connection because of the personality changes that many heart transplant patients experienced. Many recipients took on the characteristics and personality of the person who donated the heart. Research has shown that the heart communicates with the brain in several ways and can also act independently of the head brain. More recent discoveries in the area of neurocardiology have shown that the messages the heart sends the brain affect our perceptions, mental processes, feelings, and performance in profound ways.

Suggesting that there are actually three brains may seem to fly in the face of conventional medical thinking. Western medicine is primarily based on the mechanistic school of thought that sees the body as a machine made up of various interlocking parts. Mechanists take the approach that each body part and function can be understood and treated in isolation from all other parts and functions. Any new discovery that seems to shake the very foundation upon which Western medical theory is based may take years, if ever, to be accepted by more mainstream thinking. However, indigenous cultures throughout history thought these different areas of the body had their own consciousness or awareness, with heart being more powerful than the brain. It seems Western medicine is just playing catch-up with some of these more subtle but powerful integrations.

The vitalistic school of thought, which dates back to ancient Egypt, holds that life is more complex than a series of chemical reactions, and much more than the sum of its parts. Each body is animated by an organizing vital force called prana or chi that directs the body and its healing processes. Every part of the body influences the whole. This is the basis of traditional Chinese medicine, naturopathic medicine, Ayurveda, and other forms of complementary medicine. Scientific studies are now discovering that the human organism is truly a vast, multi-dimensional network of communicating systems in which mental process, emotions, and physiological systems are all intricately intertwined. Thus the interactions of the three brains have significant relevance and they must all be considered fundamental components that determine our very essence and identity, and ultimately determine our optimal mental, emotional, physical, and spiritual health.

Many people think that brain disorders are rare and that they will never be affected by them. This belief is far from accurate. In fact, the US Surgeon General reports that mental illnesses are so common that few families are untouched. My own mother suffered for years with dementia, as did my grandmother and my aunt. They also had heart-related conditions that contributed to the development of dementia. Recent research has discovered that the characteristic plaques or tangles found in the brains of people with Alzheimer's disease are also present in neurons in their guts.

However, not all neurological and mental health disorders involve the three brains. More recently and even closer to my heart, six years ago my 32-year-old son was diagnosed with an inoperable brain tumour. He is probably the smartest person I know. He received academic scholarships throughout his schooling, graduated from university with honours, and was working as an accountant at the time of his diagnosis. Within a year of being diagnosed he was unable to work due to various brain changes. However, he started on a very rigorous natural supplement program, and today his tumour is stable and he is able to work on a part-time basis.

The effects of any brain disorder are devastating for the individual as well as their loved ones. All chronic disease causes pain and suffering in different ways, but brain disorders are the only conditions that affect the core of who a person is – the very essence of their being. The individual does not change on the inside; their heart is still the same, but their ability to express themselves through their interactions with the world around them becomes more challenging. In some cases, as in people with severe dementia, it becomes impossible.

During my mother's journey with dementia, at times the pain in my heart was so great that I had to find a way to try to make things a little lighter. So I would say, "We spend our whole life learning to live in the moment and when we finally do, we call it dementia". Making light of a difficult situation helped me cope a little better at times and to see that my mom was "still there", just in a different way, and it was up to me to adjust to these changes because she couldn't.

Cognitive decline is not part of the normal process of aging, but today we are seeing increasing numbers of people with cognitive and memory problems. Therefore, it becomes even more important to know that there are many things a person can do to prevent memory decline at any age. For example, Dr. Thomas Crook, an internationally recognized memory expert who spent his career researching memory and memory loss, states that a natural supplement called phosphatidylserine (PS) can slow, halt, or reverse the decline of memory and mental function due to aging. He states, "PS is by far the best of all drugs and nutritional supplements we have ever tested for retarding age-associated memory impairment".

Even if you or a family member have not experienced a mental health disorder directly, it is very likely that you know someone who has. According to recent estimates, approximately 20% of North Americans, or about one in five people over the age of 18, suffer from a diagnosable mental health disorder in a given year. Approximately 12 million children under the age of 18 have mental disorders, and depression in adolescents may be as high as one in eight. Suicide is the third leading cause of death for 15–24-year-olds and the sixth leading cause of death for 5–15-year-olds, which is very concerning.

A variety of factors may be contributing to the increase in the number of people developing different brain disorders. Diabetes, heart disease, psychosocial stress, and other stressors including environmental toxins, electromagnetic frequencies, drugs and alcohol, brain allergens, and nutritional deficiencies all increase the risk for different three-brain disorders. The developing brain is the most sensitive to these risk factors. Scientists used to think the brain stopped developing within a few years of birth, but MRI scans of adolescent brains have revealed that not only is there major reorganization in the teenage brain, but it continues to develop until the early twenties and even early thirties.

More and more people, both young and old, are being diagnosed with brain disorders, including anxiety, depression, insomnia, schizophrenia, learning disorders, and dementias. Learning about the causes and risk factors associated with these conditions will give you a greater understanding of what you can do to help prevent and treat these life-limiting disorders. Treating people with brain disorders can be very challenging. There are a myriad of pharmaceutical medications that may help some people with their symptoms, but in many cases these medications are ineffective in the long term, and they often have unwanted and sometimes harmful side effects. Pharmaceuticals target areas of the head brain rather than taking into consideration the whole person and the interaction of the three brains in mental health. There is accumulating evidence showing that nutrients from whole foods and supplements are important modifiers of brain plasticity, helping the brain regenerate and heal. Exercise and dietary factors are effective, non-invasive ways to help counteract neurological and cognitive disorders associated with three brain imbalances.

These new discoveries in the area of neuroscience are brain changers: change your brain, change your life. *This is not an alternative approach. It is fundamental to optimal brain health.* This book is about providing solutions in order to maintain who you are, your identity. For who are you if you lose "you"?

Rather than continually waiting for "new and improved" drugs that attempt to offer better health through chemistry, let's get back to basics and start taking more responsibility for our own health and our environment. We need to learn to appreciate and respect the interconnectedness of each and every aspect of our physical, mental, emotional, and spiritual levels, and to learn to have reverence for each person and for all other living things. *We are all part of, and influenced by, the whole.*

The Three Brains: The Heart, Gut, and Head Brains

We have three brains – our head brain, our heart brain, and our gut brain. The three brains are like an orchestra, with billions of neurons cooperating to produce a harmonic symphony – harnessing together an ever-changing network of neurons that work in synchrony. Oscillations created by electrical impulses from the three brains synchronize various operations within and across the vast neuronal communication networks. Together the oscillations ensure that all components are able to do their job at the right time, the way a conductor creates order among the large number of instruments in an orchestra. In contrast, when synchronization fails, our three brains no longer function properly, leading to various mental health and neurodegenerative conditions.

The ancient Egyptians were responsible for the oldest written record of the word "brain". They also provided the first written accounts of the anatomy of the brain, the meninges (coverings of the brain) and cerebrospinal fluid. The word brain appears on an ancient paper-like document (a *papyrus*) written around the year 1700 BCE, but its usage is based on texts that go back to about 3000 BCE. However, the brain was not always held in high regard. Ancient Greek philosopher Aristotle thought intelligence was located in the heart, not the brain. In addition, even though the ancient Egyptians provided first accounts of the anatomy of the brain, they held the heart in higher regard as the centre of consciousness.

The Roles of the Three Brains

Although the head, heart, and gut brains work together, they have obvious different physical functions and they also perform different mental and emotional roles. For example, as indicated in Figure 1.1, our head brain analyzes information and applies logic. In contrast, our heart brain senses the world through emotion and feelings, and our gut brain is used for understanding our identity and who we are in the world. The gut brain also helps us learn self-preservation by teaching us to follow our instinct – the "gut feeling" we all experience at times.

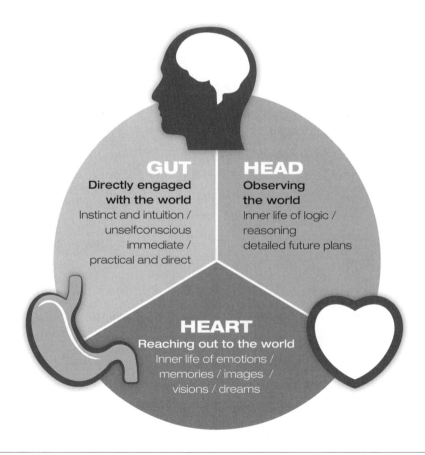

GUT
Directly engaged
with the world
Instinct and intuition /
unselfconscious
immediate /
practical and direct

HEAD
Observing
the world
Inner life of logic /
reasoning
detailed future plans

HEART
Reaching out to the world
Inner life of emotions /
memories / images /
visions / dreams

Figure 1.1 The roles of the three brains

In today's modern world, we are encouraged to focus mainly on our head brain. But we also need to use our other two brains to process our feelings and listen to our intuition to help keep us in balance.

The Head Brain

The brain is a 1.4 kg (3 lb) mass of wrinkly fatty material. In concert with the gut and heart brains, it enables you to think, learn, create, and feel emotions. The brain has been referred to as the most complex thing we have discovered so far in our universe. So the next time someone calls you a "fat" head, just say thank you and consider it a compliment!

The Brain's Electrical Impulses

The brain is awash with electrical activity. Electrical impulses create a strong electromagnetic field that is the basis for the electroencephalogram (EEG), which measures disturbances in brainwaves or oscillations as a way to diagnose various brain disorders.

The brain is composed of an estimated 100 billion neurons. Each neuron produces and transmits electrical impulses that travel from the cell body down long fibres called axons until they reach a junction, or synapse, with another neuron. At the junction point, the electrical impulses fire chemical messengers, called neurotransmitters, across the synaptic gap to receptors on the next cell. Having received the message, that neuron then generates its own electrical impulse and oscillations, commonly called brainwaves. Each neuron is simultaneously sending and receiving impulses to and from thousands of other neurons; one neuron can electrically alter millions of other neurons.

The Anatomy of the Brain

The many different areas of the brain all have different roles and functions. The area called the cerebrum is most likely to influence common mental health disorders. The cerebrum is divided into symmetrical hemispheres and each hemisphere is divided into four lobes – the frontal, parietal, temporal, and occipital lobes – each with specific functions. The neurons, or nerve cells, in each lobe produce different neurotransmitters. These neurotransmitters are the chemical messengers that communicate information throughout our brains and body by relaying signals between neurons.

The frontal lobes are considered our emotional control centre and are home to our personality or our identity. There is no other part of the brain where lesions or chemical imbalances can cause such a wide variety of mental health symptoms. The neurons in the frontal lobes produce the neurotransmitter dopamine.

The temporal lobes are involved with the processing of auditory information, visual recognition, language, learning, and memory. They are also the key to comprehending speech; we could not understand someone talking to us if it wasn't for the temporal lobes. The three most common dysfunctions of this area of the brain are Alzheimer's disease, temporal lobe epilepsy, and memory disorders. The neurotransmitter produced by neurons in the temporal lobes is gamma-aminobutyric acid (GABA), a calming neurotransmitter.

The parietal lobes are responsible for tactile perception/touch and special awareness. They integrate sensory information from various parts of the body. The neurons in the parietal lobes produce the neurotransmitter acetylcholine, a building block of myelin, which insulates and protects the neurons. Damage to the parietal lobes may result in language disorders, cognitive problems, learning disorders, and memory disorders such as Alzheimer's.

The occipital lobes are the centre of our visual perception system. Visual memory is the ability to retain information about colours, our environment, shapes, faces, etc. Common symptoms of the occipital lobe dysfunction include lack of rational thinking, short-term memory loss, visual changes, or sleep problems. The neurons in the occipital lobes produce the neurotransmitter serotonin.

Neurotransmitters – The Head-Brain's Messengers

The brain uses neurotransmitters to tell our heart to beat, our lungs to breathe, and our stomach to digest. Neurotransmitters can affect mood, sleep, concentration, and weight, and can cause adverse mental and emotional symptoms when they are out of balance. Neurotransmitters are also found in the gut brain and heart brain. It is estimated that 86% of North Americans have suboptimal neurotransmitter levels. Neurotransmitter levels can be depleted in many ways: stress, poor diet, neurotoxins, genetic predisposition, drugs (prescription and recreational), alcohol, and caffeine can cause imbalances in the brain's neurotransmitters.

There are two kinds of neurotransmitters, inhibitory and excitatory. Excitatory neurotransmitters stimulate the brain, and those that calm the brain and help create balance are called inhibitory. Inhibitory neurotransmitters balance mood and are easily depleted when the excitatory neurotransmitters are overactive. The most recognized neurotransmitters in the head brain include serotonin, GABA, taurine, dopamine, norepinephrine, epinephrine, glutamate, and acetylcholine.

Inhibitory neurotransmitters

Serotonin

Serotonin is most commonly believed to be a neurotransmitter, although some consider it to be a hormone. It is responsible for maintaining mood balance, appetite and digestion, sleep, memory, and sexual desire and function. Serotonin also regulates other processes such as carbohydrate cravings and pain control, and low levels are associated with decreased immune system function. Serotonin is manufactured in the head brain and the gut brain. The majority of the body's serotonin, approximately 90–95%, can be found in the gastrointestinal tract, confirming another link between the gut and what we currently consider "brain" disorders.

Commonly prescribed antidepressant medications (called selective serotonin reuptake inhibitors or SSRIs) increase serotonin levels, so it is little wonder that medications meant to cause chemical changes in the mind often provoke gastrointestinal issues as a side effect. Irritable bowel syndrome, which afflicts more than two million North Americans, also results, in part, from too much serotonin in the gut, and could perhaps be regarded as a mental disorder of the gut brain. Scientists remain uncertain of whether decreased levels of serotonin contribute to depression, or if depression causes a decrease in serotonin.

GABA

The main inhibitory neurotransmitter in the brain is GABA, and its primary role is to calm the brain, slow things down, and relax individuals. It acts like a brake in the central nervous system (CNS). Insufficient levels of GABA result in nervousness, anxiety and panic disorders, and aggressive behaviour. Other effects of low levels of GABA include decreased eye contact and anti-social behaviour, as seen in children with autism spectrum disorder and attention deficit problems or in people with anxiety or chronic pain syndromes. Maintaining sufficient levels of GABA is crucial when treating these conditions.

Low levels of GABA also play a role in alcoholism, drug addiction, and cravings for sugar and carbohydrates, as these substances will temporarily and artificially increase GABA. As a result, individuals are unconsciously drawn to these substances. However, these substances also deplete neurotransmitters, so they simply compound the problem.

Taurine as a neurotransmitter

Taurine is a sulphur-containing amino acid considered to be a powerful inhibitory neurotransmitter in the CNS. It is used to calm excitable tissues such as the heart, skeletal muscles, and the brain. Taurine plays a central role in CNS development by maintaining the structural integrity of the membrane, regulating calcium transport, and maintaining homeostasis. Taurine also protects against glutamate-induced cell damage. It is believed that taurine is neuroprotective due to its role as an antioxidant.

Excitatory neurotransmitters

Dopamine

Dopamine is a neurotransmitter that influences memory, pleasure and reward, behaviour and cognition, attention, sleep, and mood and learning. Dopamine is very important in the reward system whereby we feel pleasure, achieve heightened arousal, and do much of our learning. It also helps with focus, concentration, and memory, as well as motivation. Conditions associated with dysfunctions in the dopamine system include Parkinson's disease, schizophrenia, restless leg syndrome, and attention deficit hyperactivity disorder (ADHD).

A wide variety of highly addictive drugs, including cocaine and methamphetamine (speed), as well as prescription stimulant drugs commonly prescribed for ADHD (e.g., Ritalin, Adderall, Dexedrine), act directly on the dopamine/norepinephrine system. Dopamine is considered to be both excitatory and inhibitory.

Norepinephrine and epinephrine

Norepinephrine, along with epinephrine (adrenaline), is responsible for the "fight-or-flight" response to stress, which causes increased heart rate, blood sugar, and blood flow to the muscles in response to a perceived or real threat. Chronic stress can cause imbalances in these neurotransmitters, resulting in anxiety, low energy, mood disorders, ADHD, and sleep disorders.

Glutamate

Glutamate is one of the most abundant neurotransmitters in the body, but particularly in the nervous system and the brain. It is the brain's main excitatory neurotransmitter. Through a complex series of pathways, glutamate is a precursor for GABA, the brain's main inhibitory neurotransmitter.

The glutamate receptors are important for communication between brain cells, memory formation, learning, and general regulation. Excess glutamate can contribute to disorders such as autism, Parkinson's disease, amyotrophic lateral sclerosis (ALS), fibromyalgia, multiple sclerosis, insomnia, hyperactivity, ADHD, obsessive compulsive disorder (OCD), and anxiety disorders. It is also thought to be associated with Alzheimer's.

Acetylcholine

Acetylcholine is the most common neurotransmitter, with important responsibilities in the entire nervous system. In the CNS (brain and spinal cord), acetylcholine modulates communications regarding arousal, reward, learning, attention, and responsiveness to sensory stimuli. In the peripheral nervous system, acetylcholine is responsible for activating muscle movement and helps modulate heartbeat, among other things. Damage or disruption to the acetylcholine-producing system has been shown to be associated with the memory deficits, including Alzheimer's.

The Blood-Brain Barrier

The brain's circulatory system consists of 644 km (400 miles) of blood vessels that nourish the brain. The brain is protected from toxins by the blood-brain barrier (BBB), a filtering mechanism of the capillaries that carry blood to the brain, and the brain's first line of defence. The second line of defence is the microglia, the brain's white blood cells, which are key players in the immune response to infection or foreign invaders. However, when the microglia are activated by injury, infection, or other BBB "busters", they release inflammatory chemicals, causing further damage to the protective barrier.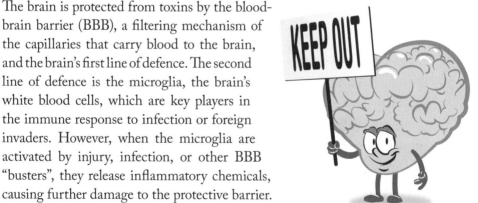

The BBB is impermeable, for the most part letting in only glucose, oxygen, and other nutrients that brain cells need to function. This prevents most of the toxins and infectious agents we encounter daily from coming into contact with our brain's delicate microenvironment. As a result, the brain's balance of electrolytes is preserved, such as potassium, which if disturbed can wreak havoc on the electrical signalling required for normal brain function. When the barrier gets damaged, however, dangerous molecules and immune cells that are not supposed to be there can slip inside.

Blood-brain barrier busters

Several factors can break down the brain's defensive wall and cause BBB permeability or a "leaky" brain, including:

- Hypertension
- Inflammatory responses associated with brain surgeries, radiation, traumatic brain injury, and concussions
- Microbes including viral (e.g., influenza, CMV, Coxsacki, H5N1, Guillain-Barre, Herpes simplex, HIV) or bacterial (e.g., streptococcus, *Chlamydia pneumoniae*), moulds, and mycotoxins
- Electromagnetic frequencies (EMFs) from power lines, computers, cell phones, and microwaves, along with radiation
- Environmental toxins such as chemicals, insecticides, pesticides, solvents (e.g., benzene), and cigarette smoke
- A faulty gut-brain axis, including dysbiosis (an imbalance in gut bacteria), endotoxins from bacterial overgrowth, and PCBs and other toxins ingested from food or water
- Other exposures such as toxic metals (e.g., aluminum, mercury), certain medications, shock, stress, food allergens (e.g., gluten, dairy), and inflammation

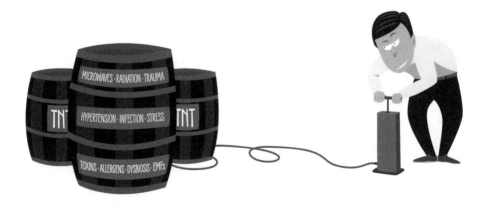

When the BBB becomes more permeable, the foreign invaders can potentially cause harm to the delicate neurological tissues. Damage to this protective barrier, which results in a leaky brain, is an underappreciated cause of many mental health, neurological, and autoimmune disorders, including:

- Learning disorders such as ADHD, attention deficit disorder (ADD), autism spectrum disorders, and developmental disorders
- Mental health disorders such as anxiety, depression, sleep disorders, cognitive disorders, memory problems, OCD, and schizophrenia
- Neurodegenerative disorders and diseases of aging, including senile dementia, Alzheimer's, epilepsy, multiple sclerosis, Parkinson's disease, stroke, and peripheral neuropathy

According to current thinking in Western medicine, the brain is thought to be the central command post for the rest of the body. However, new discoveries are always being made to replace current thinking. New evidence shows a direct correlation between both the gut and the brain, and the heart and the brain.

The head brain has been studied for centuries. As a result, the information available is vast in comparison to the modes of function and the anatomy of the gut and heart brains.

The Gut Brain – Neurogastroenterology

For hundreds of years, people have believed that the gut interacts with the brain to influence health and disease. An original pioneer in this field was Dr. Byron Robinson, who published The Abdominal and Pelvic Brain in 1907. However, this concept was later abandoned as a superstition by scientific medicine. The idea of a gut brain was rediscovered by more contemporary neuroscientists in the 1990s when the field of neurogastroenterology was born.

An increasing amount of evidence has shown that gut microbiota play a role in the function of the CNS (brain and spinal cord) through metabolic, endocrine (hormone), and immune pathways. In particular, studies have shown an association between gut flora composition and mood disorders, as well as cognitive processes such as learning and memory. Gut microbiota additionally contribute to the early development of normal social and cognitive behaviours, and in older age have an impact on brain plasticity and cognitive function.

The Anatomy of the Gut Brain

When you look at the anatomy of the human body, you can't fail to notice the brain and its offshoots of nerve cells running along the spinal cord. The enteric nervous system (ENS), or gut brain, is far less obvious, which is why it wasn't discovered until the mid-nineteenth century. The gut brain is embedded in the wall of the digestive system and has long been known to control digestion. It is also the original nervous system, emerging in the first vertebrates over 500 million years ago. It became more complex as vertebrates evolved – possibly even giving rise to the brain itself.

The gut brain shares many features with the head brain. It is made up of various types of neurons with glial cells that provide support and protection for neurons in the CNS and peripheral nervous system. The gut brain also has its own version of a BBB to keep its physiological environment stable.

The gut brain can work both independently of and in conjunction with the head brain. Although you may not be conscious of your gut "thinking", many people are aware of and have learned to follow a feeling in the gut called "gut instinct".

Gut-Brain Neurotransmitters

The gut brain is a centre point of the nervous system, hormonal system, and immune system. It is also responsible for the balance and regulation of our neurotransmitters. According to Candace B. Pert, PhD, formerly chief of brain biochemistry at the National Institutes of Health (NIH), neurotransmitters are our molecules of emotion and, as a result, they are important players in mood regulation.

The neurotransmitters in the gut have not been thoroughly studied, but new information is constantly emerging. The gut brain produces a wide range of hormones and around 40 neurotransmitters of the same classes as those found in the head brain. In fact, neurons in the gut are thought to generate as much dopamine as the brain and about 90–95% of the serotonin.

In the brain, dopamine is known as the feel-good neurotransmitter and is associated with the pleasure and the reward system. It acts the same way in the gut. Dopamine also transmits messages between neurons and is involved in preventing depression and regulating moods, sleep, appetite, and body temperature.

Serotonin produced in the gut also gets into the blood, where it is involved in repairing damaged cells in the liver and lungs. It is important for normal development of the heart, as well as regulating bone density. Serotonin in the gut is also crucial for the proper development of the gut brain. Serotonin-producing cells develop early on, and if this development is affected by infection or extreme stress at a young age, the gut brain cannot form properly. Later in life this could lead to irritable bowel syndrome, which is often accompanied by depression. Serotonin seeping from the gut brain might even play some part in autism, which could explain why so many children with autism have intestinal abnormalities in addition to elevated levels of gut-produced serotonin in their blood due to "leaky gut".

The Gut-Brain Barrier

The gut barrier shares many of the same functions as the BBB. It stops potentially dangerous invaders, such toxins, bacteria, and viruses, from getting inside the body. If a pathogen should cross the gut lining, immune cells in the gut wall secrete inflammatory substances that are detected by neurons in the gut brain. The gut brain then initiates diarrhea, vomiting, or both. Inflammation also causes leaky gut, as described in Chapter 2.

Gut Microbiome

New research shows that gut bacteria communicate with and influence brain function. An imbalance in the good and bad gut microbiota, called dysbio-sis, is associated with a number of brain disorders and symptoms, including ADHD, autism, OCD, mood swings, memory and cognition problems, anxiety, depression, and insomnia, as well as neurological disorders such as Parkinson's and Alzheimer's.

In Parkinson's, for example, the problems with movement and muscle control are caused by a loss of dopamine-producing cells in the brain. However, research at the University of Frankfurt, Germany, has found that the protein clumps that do the damage, called Lewy bodies, are also present in dopamine-producing neurons in the gut. In fact, based on the distribution of Lewy bodies in people who died of Parkinson's, scientists think the disease actually starts in the gut. Similarly, the characteristic plaques or tangles found in the brains of people with Alzheimer's are also present in neurons in their guts.

Our senses, behaviour, and intelligence emerge in part from electrical com-munications among neurons in the head brain. Scientists have found that like neurons in the head brain, bacteria communities (microbiome) in the gut communicate with each other through electrical signals. This research was headed by Gürol Süel, PhD, an associate professor of molecular biology at the

University of California, who stated "Our discovery not only changes the way we think about bacteria, but also how we think about our brain."

Such gut-to-brain signals may also explain why fatty foods make us feel good. When ingested, fatty acids are detected by cell receptors in the lining of the gut, which send nerve signals to the brain. Brain scans of volunteers given fatty acids directly into the gut had a lower response to pictures and music designed to make them feel sad compared to those given saline. They also reported feeling only about half as sad as the other group.

MICROBES AND BEHAVIOUR

In a study published in the journal *Gastroenterology* in 2011, researchers from McMaster University gave typically timid mice a mixture of antibiotics that changed the composition of their gut bacteria. The researchers recorded a striking change in their behaviour: the mice became bold and adventurous. In a follow-up experiment, the same researchers took bacteria from the guts of the shy mice and swapped it with bacteria from the guts of mice known for their brave behaviour. They also placed the gut bacteria from the brave mice into the guts of the shy, nervous mice. The result was remarkable. The normally nervous mice became more fearless explorers, while the typically venturesome mice grew more timid and shy. The influence of the gut bacteria *overcame* the genetic predisposition of the mice. The scientists were astounded!

These new discoveries about how the gut brain is implicated in many different health disorders means the gut-brain axis deserves a lot more recognition than it has had in the past.

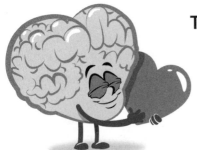

The Heart Brain – Neurocardiology

We are usually taught that the heart is a pump and its sole purpose is to propel blood throughout the body. However, when physicists did a study on the vessels of the heart and their links, they found that in order to pump blood around the body, the heart would have to be capable of shooting a 45 kg (100 lb) weight over a kilometre high in the air, which of course it cannot do. The researchers discovered that the blood moves counterintuitively of its own accord around the body, and the heart plays a much more subtle role in stabilizing that pumping motion.

The heart brain, like the gut brain, communicates with the head brain via nerve fibres running through the vagus nerve and the spinal column. However, more recent discoveries in the area of neurocardiology have found other communication networks between the heart and brain. The heart brain contains around 40,000 neurons that communicate with the brain. The heart also stores memories much like the brain does; it has neurotransmitters and neurons, just like the brain, that are connected by synapses. Experiments have demonstrated that the signals continuously sent from the heart to the brain influence brain centres involved with cognition, emotional processing, and perception.

The Heart Brain's Electrical Impulses

In addition to the complex and extensive neural communication network linking the heart and brain, the two brains also communicate via electromagnetic field (EMF) interactions. Like the head brain, the heart brain is a powerful electromagnetic generator and receiver. All organisms have unique electromagnetic signatures, and the heart is able to perceive these EMFs, which are then routed to the brain for analysis.

The heart brain's EMF is 60 times greater in amplitude than in the head brain, and the magnetic component is approximately 5,000 times stronger. The heart's rhythmic field has a powerful influence throughout the body, and research indicates that the brain's rhythms naturally synchronize to the heart's rhythms. The rate of our heartbeat, or its contraction, changes depending on our emotions. For example, during sustained positive emotions such as love or appreciation, our blood pressure and respiratory rhythms adjust to match the heart's rhythm. Research done at the HeartMath Institute in California suggests that the heart's field acts as a carrier wave for information that provides a synchronizing signal for the entire body.

Heart-Brain Hormones and Neurotransmitters

The heart was reclassified as an endocrine gland in 1983, when a hormone produced and released by the heart called atrial natriuretic factor (ANF) was isolated. This hormone exerts its effect on the blood vessels, kidneys, adrenal glands, and a large number of regulatory regions in the brain. It was also found that the heart contains cells that release the neurotransmitters noradrenaline and dopamine, which were once thought to be produced only by neurons in the head brain.

More recently, researchers discovered that similar to the pituitary gland, the heart also secretes oxytocin, commonly referred to as the "love" hormone. In addition to its functions in childbirth and lactation, recent evidence indicates that this hormone is also involved in cognition, tolerance, adaptation, and sexual and social behaviours. Concentrations of oxytocin in the heart were found to be as high as those found in the brain.

Researchers have found that oxytocin is beneficial for many mental health conditions, including social anxieties, depression and other mood disorders, post-traumatic stress, and autism spectrum disorders. In addition, it has proven beneficial in reducing stressed-induced cortisol levels and helping with weight loss by balancing metabolism and reducing glucose intolerance and insulin resistance. Interestingly, oxytocin and the oxytocin receptors have also been found in the intestinal tract, where they improve gut motility and decrease intestinal inflammation.

The heart is a much more complex organ, both of perception and cognition, than we had previously been led to believe. Recently, scientists have also discovered that the heart is involved in the processing and decoding of intuitive information. In fact, tests have shown that the heart appears to receive intuitive information before the brain does. This could be the basis for the saying, "follow your heart and you will never go wrong".

The Heart Brain and the Gut Microbiome

Prebiotics and probiotics support the heart brain as well as the head brain. Prebiotics are specialized plant fibres that nourish the good bacteria already in the large bowel or colon, while probiotics introduce good bacteria into the gut. It has been shown that prebiotics lower associated risk factors for atherosclerotic cardiovascular disease when associated with elevated insulin and triglycerides.

Probiotic bacteria, particularly bifidobacteria and some lactobacilli strains, tend to lower production of proinflammatory cytokines. This means less inflammation and less chance of accumulation of cholesterol in the area. Probiotics also help reduce blood cholesterol production through different mechanisms, and probiotic bacteria have been shown to break down cholesterol and use it for nourishment.

Inflammation is now recognized as one of the main contributing factors to heart disease, including chronic heart failure. Pro-inflammatory cytokines appear to play important roles in these diseases. Disturbances in the gut-brain barrier trigger cytokine generation, causing inflammation and leading to cardiovascular problems. It goes both ways – disturbances in heart function can lead to a disruption in the gut-brain barrier, which amplifies the inflammatory response.

The Gut-Heart-Brain Axis

The head brain has been studied for centuries, and as a result, we have much more information about how scientists think it works compared to the heart and gut brains. However, in recent years the intricate workings of the other two brains has peaked the interest of many researchers. Over time, we will begin to see more and more information about the unique workings of the heart and gut brains. Figure 1.2 summarizes some of the functions, interactions, and similarities of the three brains.

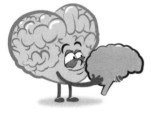 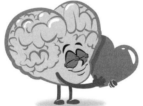 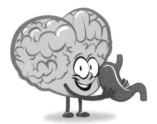

BRAIN	HEART	GUT
• Glial cell support • 85 billion neurons • 100 neurotransmitters identified • 5–10% of body's serotonin • 50% of body's dopamine • Blood-brain barrier protects from toxins • Communicates with other brains via vagus nerve, spinal cord, neurotransmitters, and EMFs	• Hormones and neurotransmitters similar to head brain • Communicates with other brains via vagus nerve and spinal cord, peptides, nerve impulses, hormones, neurotransmitters, and EMFs • Electromagnetic field is 60 times greater than the brain • Magnetic component is 5,000 times stronger than the brain and affects every cell in the body • Has its own nervous system and can act independently	• Glial cell support • 50 million neurons • 40 neurotransmitters identified • 50% of body's dopamine • 90–95% of body's serotonin • Protective barrier to protect from toxins • Communicates with other brains via vagus nerve, microflora (gut bacteria) • Can act independently

Figure 1.2 Three-brain similarities and interactions

Keeping the Three Brains Healthy

A healthy diet and exercise are the foundation for optimal health on all levels. In today's world, with added exposure to toxins, increased stress, and decreased nutrients in our soils, it becomes even more important to supplement our lifestyle with added vitamins, minerals, essential fatty acids, and botanicals. The supplements mentioned below are some of the most important nutrients to keep the three brains functioning optimally.

Key Supplements for the Three Brains

In addition to a good quality multivitamin and mineral, many supplements play a role in maintaining optimal brain nutrition. While many nutrients are discussed throughout this book, the following supplements can be considered the foundation for supporting the three brains.

Ginkgo biloba

Ginkgo increases blood flow to the brain and enhances memory concentration, mental clarity, and learning abilities. The antioxidant properties of gingko have been found to inhibit beta-amyloid plaques in Alzheimer's. Gingko has also been shown to lower the risk of atherosclerosis and heart attack. It supports the head and heart brains.

Dosage: 150–250 mg daily of a standardized extract.

Note: Contraindicated in people taking blood thinners such as Coumadin.

Phosphatidylserine (PS)

PS is an important phospholipid that can enhance mood and memory ability and protect from age-related memory decline and dementias, including Alzheimer's. PS supports the head brain. For more information on PS, refer to Chapter 5.

Dosage: 100–300 mg daily.

Pyrroloquinoline quinone (PQQ)

PQQ provides a wide range of benefits for healthy brain function, including antioxidant support and protection against the damaging effects of neurotoxins. Overall, PQQ helps prevent memory problems and cognitive decline, and has been shown to decrease myocardial infarct size and improve cardiac function. PQQ supports the head and heart brains. Refer to Chapter 9 for more information on PQQ.

Dosage: 20 mg daily.

Curcumin

Curcumin has potent antioxidant and anti-inflammatory properties that can help prevent and support the inflammatory cause of depression and other mood disorders and cognitive decline. Curcumin has also demonstrated a significant role in the treatment of dementias, including Alzheimer's. Inflammation is one of the main factors in cardiovascular and intestinal disorders as well. Curcumin supports the three brains. Refer to Chapters 3 and 9 for more information on curcumin.

Dosage: 300 mg daily of a brand that has been optimized for maximum absorption.

Fish oil

Omega-3 fatty acids are found in cold water fish and are involved in the synthesis of neurotransmitters. They are highly concentrated in the brain and deficiencies have been linked to memory and cognitive problems, as well as dementias. Fish oils have anti-inflammatory effects and are beneficial for heart, gut, and brain health. Refer to Chapter 5 for more information on the importance of fish oils for brain health.

Dosage: 1000–3000 mg daily.

CoQ10

Hypertension damages brain structures and leads to reduced cognitive ability and a greater risk for dementias. CoQ10 supports cardiovascular function and helps regulate blood pressure. It supports head and heart brains. Refer to Chapter 5 for more information on how cardiovascular health affects cognitive ability and memory.

Dosage: 50–150 mg daily.

Lutein

Although lutein is better known for its role in eye health, evidence now indicates that lutein may be important for brain function as well. The brain is vulnerable to free radical damage due to its relatively low antioxidant levels and high concentration of fatty acids. Lutein functions as both an antioxidant and an anti-inflammatory agent and is therefore beneficial for those conditions where inflammation is a contributing cause, such as depression, memory problems, cognitive disorders, cardiovascular problems, and intestinal inflammation. Lutein supports the three brains.

Dosage: 10–20 mg daily.

Magnesium

Every single cell in the human body demands adequate magnesium to function, or it will perish. Magnesium is commonly deficient in our soils, and up to 35% of Canadians have an intake below the average requirement. Soft tissue containing the highest concentrations of magnesium in the body include the brain and the heart, two organs that produce a large amount of electrical activity and that can be especially vulnerable to magnesium insufficiency. Magnesium works in concert with calcium to regulate electrical impulses in the cells. It supports the three brains.

Dosage: 400–800 mg daily (bisglycinate form of magnesium).

Vitamin D

Scientists have now linked this fat-soluble nutrient's hormone-like activity to a number of functions throughout the body. Vitamin D is involved in neurotransmitter synthesis and nerve growth, as well as protecting neurons and reducing inflammation. Vitamin D deficiency is a risk factor for cardiovascular disease, cognitive problems, and dementias, and emerging evidence suggests that the vitamin D pathway may be important for communication between the microbiota in the gut. It supports the three brains.

Dosage: 3000–5000 IU daily.

Grapeseed extract

Grapeseed contains proanthocyanidin complexes, which are powerful antioxidants that destroy free radicals. Free radicals damage DNA and cause cell death. This contributes to aging as well as to the development of a number of health problems, including heart disease and memory decline. Grapeseed extract supports the three brains.

Dosage: 400 mg daily of an extract standardized to 80% oligomeric proanthocyanidins.

Prebiotics and Probiotics

Prebiotics are specialized plant fibres that nourish the good bacteria already in the large bowel or colon, while probiotics introduce good bacteria into the gut. Many studies confirm the benefits of fibre and probiotics for the prevention and treatment of mental health and neurological disorders, lowering cardiovascular risk factors, and many intestinal disorders. Prebiotics and probiotics support the three brains. A strain such as BB536 contains *Bifidobacterium longum*, the most prevalent bacteria in the intestine.

Dosage: 1–2 capsules daily.

 LOOK for a product such as...

Rather than purchasing each of the above-mentioned products individually, some brands offer a comprehensive "kit" that includes the most essential supplements for brain health in convenient daily packets. For example, **Daily Brain** includes phosphatidylserine-enriched sunflower (containing naturally occurring phosphatidylcholine [PC], phosphatidylinositol [PI], and phosphatidylethanolamine [PE]), curcumin, omega-3 fatty acids EPA and DHA, grapeseed extract, and key probiotic strains.

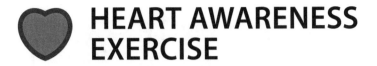

HEART AWARENESS EXERCISE

Look at everything that you encounter in your life. Just look at it. Allow yourself to notice how it appears visually, then ask yourself, how does it feel? In that moment, that conscious action will focus attention on the electromagnetic signature coming from the heart. See what feeling you experience. You may not have a name for it, but just feel it; experience it.

Because we do not consciously focus on the heart when it comes to listening to our feelings, you may not be able to articulate how you feel. This exercise can help open up the realm of perception through the heart. You will learn to trust and follow your heart. Listen to yourself to see what you are saying. Do you say "I think…" or "I feel…" or "My gut says…"? You can learn to recognize which "mind" you are using.

The shift away from the belief that the brain is the only seat of consciousness is a very big step. But consciousness or human awareness is throughout the body, and can shift to any area of biological electromagnetic oscillations in the body. The brain, the heart, and the gut are the three primary areas, and perception will depend on which location is most active.

Different indigenous cultures throughout history believed these different areas of the body had their own consciousness or awareness, with the heart being more powerful than the brain. Western medicine is just starting to consider many of these more subtle, but powerful, integrations.

Because Western men in particular have been trained to pay attention to the brain and not the heart, they may have lost the capacity to really feel those things that are presented to their other senses. But if we start to pay more attention to how things feel and the exchange of energy, the heart begins to be reactivated as an organ of perception, rather than being seen as just a pump.

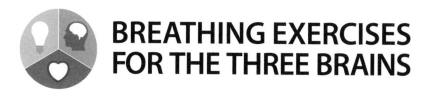 # BREATHING EXERCISES FOR THE THREE BRAINS

Become familiar with your three brains by spending a few minutes every day sitting quietly. Close your eyes and breathe into each area to activate each of the three brains. Start by breathing deeply 3–6 times into your head, then move down to your chest, and finally to your lower abdomen (just below your belly button). You don't need to do anything; just close your eyes, breathe, and notice what happens as you bring your attention into each area of the three brains.

This exercise will help you to look internally for your own answers as opposed to looking outside of yourself to others for what is right for you. With practice, you will begin to trust your own thoughts and feelings.

Focus on a problem you are experiencing right now in your life or a decision you need to make, and then begin breathing into each of your three brains:

- **As you breathe into your head, ask yourself:**
  What do I think about this situation?

- **As you breathe into your chest, ask yourself:**
  How do I feel about this situation?

- **As you breathe into your belly, ask yourself:**
  What are my gut instincts or inner voice telling me to do?

Write down the answers or insights you come up with, then follow through with what feels right for you.

Use your thinking brain and words to express your feelings and inner voice (intuition) in a respectful and honest way with the people in your life. Listen to your heart and how you really feel. Honour your feelings by expressing or saying what feels right for you. Listen to your gut instincts and learn to trust your inner voice, then act on what are good choices for you to make in life.

The information on the three brains provided in this chapter shows us how each brain works in similar ways, working independently and/or together to help maintain physical and mental emotional health.

Stress and the Three Brains

Medical research suggests that up to 90% of all illness and disease is stress-related. – Centers for Disease Control and Prevention

Chronic stress increases the risk of developing health problems, including obesity, metabolic syndrome, diabetes, heart disease, chronic inflammatory disorders, cancer, and a weakened immune system. Chronic stress also affects mental health. Many studies show a correlation between stress and the development of mood disorders, sleep disorders, obsessive compulsive disorder (OCD), dementias (including Alzheimer's disease), drug and alcohol abuse, learning problems, anxiety disorders, and depression.

Overview of Stress and Stressors

People experience stress when they perceive that there is an imbalance between demands made of them and the resources they have available to cope with those demands. Stressors are events or situations that require the body to adapt and respond in order to maintain balance or homeostasis. They include:

- **Physical** – chronic infection, illness, and pain
- **Mental and emotional** – money, work, the economy, personal relationships, family responsibilities, and family health problems
- **Lifestyle** – lack of exercise, too much sitting
- **Diet and nutrition** – depletion of the nutritional content of most foods due to modern agricultural and food processing practices; prevalence of junk food and highly processed foods in supermarkets; contamination of the soil and water supply by pollutants

- **Electromagnetic fields (EMFs)** – cell and cordless phones, microwaves, baby monitors, cell phone towers, computers, etc.

- **Environmental toxins** – heavy metals such as mercury, lead, and aluminum; pesticides and herbicides; and plastic by-products like bisphenol A and phthalates, to name a few

Some stress is absolutely normal and necessary in living creatures. We all have a built-in gauge that helps us control our reaction to various stressors. However, in today's fast-paced society, the vast majority of individuals are under a barrage of constant stressors. While some of the initial fight-or-flight stress responses may be beneficial to survival (acute stress), there is an increased risk of various physical and psychological health challenges when the stressors are prolonged (chronic stress). Stress is not something new, and it is not going away.

We will all benefit from reducing the stressors in our lives, but the obvious benefits will vary depending on our overall stress resistance capabilities. Often the stressors can be non-specific and less obvious, and we may not be aware of the effects on our bodies and minds.

The Brain "On Stress"

The Role of Hormones

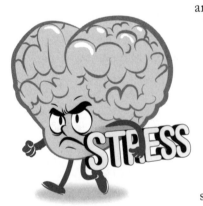

If there is a central command post for the body's stress response, it is the hypothalamus, a primitive area of the brain. Through an intricate array of hormonal signals, the hypothalamus directly connects to the pituitary gland and the main stress-reactive glands in the body, the adrenal glands. During a normal stress response, these hormones are carefully regulated to control everything from our immune system to our cardiovascular, gastrointestinal, and behavioural systems. Even minute changes in any of these levels of hormones can have a significant effect on our health.

The hypothalamus-pituitary-adrenal axis (HPA) triggers the production and release of stress hormones during acute stress reactions (fight or flight), namely epinephrine and norepinephrine. The HPA also releases cortisol, the main stress hormone, during times of chronic stress. These stress hormones travel through the bloodstream and cross the blood-brain barrier (BBB), directly and indirectly affecting brain chemistry balance.

The loss of complex thought processing during stressful events may have once allowed more primitive behaviours to take precedence in order to aid survival. However, we are no longer seeking the safety of caves while running from wild boars. Today, non-life-threatening stressors can activate these same stress response circuits, causing scattered thought, loss of focus, and judgment errors that can be detrimental to daily life, and in extreme cases, lead to mental health problems.

Over time, stressful events can lead to significant imbalances in the delicate brain chemistry, resulting in mental disorders including depression, anxiety, insomnia, post-traumatic stress disorder (PTSD), schizophrenia, and attention deficit/hyperactivity disorder (ADD, ADHD), to name a few.

Stress and the Heart Brain

The Role of Inflammation

Many traditional cultures consider the heart to be the seat of the human spirit. The age-old wisdom that it is possible to die of a broken heart is now called stress cardiomyopathy, which is also referred to as "broken heart syndrome". It is a condition in which intense emotional or physical stress can cause rapid and severe heart muscle weakness (cardiomyopathy). This condition can occur following emotional stressors such as grief, fear, extreme anger, or surprise. It can also occur following physical stressors such as stroke, seizure, difficulty breathing, or significant bleeding. In addition, scientists are finding that depression is an independent risk factor for the development of both coronary artery disease and stroke.

Stress hormones are powerful anti-inflammatory agents. However, in chronic stress, the overproduction of cortisol causes an increase in cytokines (proteins that affect the behaviour of other cells), leading to increased inflammation. Several studies have shown that increased cortisol is associated with glucose intolerance, hypertension, obesity, dyslipidemia, and elevated triglycerides and blood pressure.

It is clear that stress-induced inflammation can create significant damage to the heart brain by increasing the risk of coronary artery disease, elevating blood pressure, increasing atherosclerosis, and increasing the risk of myocardial infarction.

The Role of Emotions

The Mayo Clinic reported that psychological health is the strongest risk factor for future cardiac events in individuals with existing coronary artery disease. When researchers interviewed heart attack survivors, they found the intensity and timing of stressful emotions like anger, anxiety, and worry dramatically increased their risk. A full 50% (with some sources claiming as high as 75%) of all heart attacks occur in people without any traditional risk factors. However, people who are prone to anger, hostility, and depressive symptoms respond to stress with increased production of the stress hormones that activate the inflammatory arm of the immune system. This causes chronic inflammation, characterized by high levels of C-reactive protein (CRP.) The study showed that those people prone to anger had 2–3 times higher CRP levels than their calmer counterparts. The more pronounced their negative moods, the higher the CRP.

Stress and the Gut Brain

The Role of Microbiota

The gut-brain/head-brain axis is a two-way communication system between the central nervous system (CNS) (brain and spinal cord) and the gastrointestinal tract, as shown in Figure 2.1. Gut microbiota are the microorganisms living in the gut; collectively these microbes are called the microbiome. Alterations in the balance of gut microbiota have been linked to a broad range of diseases, including autoimmune, metabolic, and gastrointestinal disorders, and brain disorders such as depression, mood disorders, learning disorders, schizophrenia, and autism spectrum disorders.

Microbial communities within the gut are relatively resistant to change. However, it is recognized that factors such as alterations in diet, inflammation, and the administration of antibiotics can cause modifications to the microbial balance. Studies have demonstrated that psychosocial stressors can also cause alterations in the gut microbial community that can cause neurological and mental health disorders.

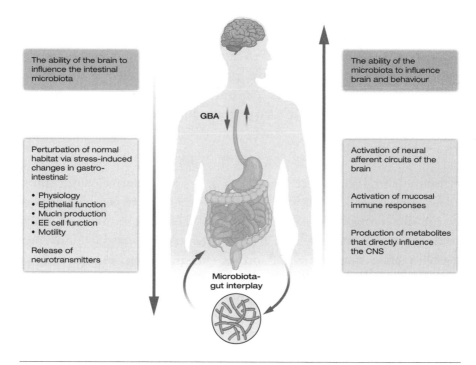

The ability of the brain to influence the intestinal microbiota

The ability of the microbiota to influence brain and behaviour

GBA

Perturbation of normal habitat via stress-induced changes in gastro-intestinal:

• Physiology
• Epithelial function
• Mucin production
• EE cell function
• Motility

Release of neurotransmitters

Activation of neural afferent circuits of the brain

Activation of mucosal immune responses

Production of metabolites that directly influence the CNS

Microbiota-gut interplay

Figure 2.1 Interaction between the gut and the brain

Research shows the role of the gut-brain/head-brain axis is to monitor and integrate gut functions, as well as to link the emotional and cognitive centres of the brain. This two-way communication network between the brain and the gut also involves the HPA axis. The HPA axis is considered the core stress axis responsible for the adaptive responses to stressors of any kind. It is a part of the limbic system, an area of the brain predominantly involved in memory and emotional responses.

It is well know that exposure to stress results in alterations to gut-brain interactions, ultimately leading to the development of a number of gastro-intestinal disorders including inflammatory bowel disease (IBD), irritable bowel syndrome (IBS), adverse food allergy-related responses, peptic ulcer, and gastroesophageal reflux disease (GERD). However, what is not commonly recognized is that it works both ways. Studies demonstrate that gut microbiota influence stress reactions and anxiety-like behaviour by directly affecting the HPA activity and the release of stress hormones, namely cortisol and epinephrine. When the gut is recolonized with healthy gut bacteria, it leads to a normalization of the HPA axis and a reversal of the exaggerated stress hormone response.

Research has shown that gut microbial imbalances alter mood and behaviour due to altered levels of brain-derived neurotrophic factor (BDNF). BDNF is one of the most important factors involved in memory, cognitive functions, muscle repair, and regeneration. For example, when animals that showed anxiety-like behaviour were treated to a 10-day course of the beneficial microbes in the form of *Bifidobacterium longum*, their behaviour normalized, as did their BDNF levels.

The "Leaky Gut" Factor

Stress can also directly affect microbiota by altering intestinal permeability, allowing bacterial antigens and other toxic substances to penetrate the gut barrier. The mucosal gut barrier is said to be the body's second skin, which serves as the first line of defence against pathogens. Increased intestinal permeability, often called "leaky gut", occurs when this protective barrier fails to prevent potentially harmful molecules from entering the bloodstream. These molecules can cause an inflammatory response, leading to brain degeneration and mood changes.

A healthy microbiome works to boost mood by generating healthy levels of brain-derived neurotrophic factor and the neurotransmitter gamma-amino-butyric acid (GABA), and by enhancing brain receptors for GABA. GABA is known to calm areas of the brain that are overactive in anxiety and panic, and in some forms of depression.

Research findings provide evidence of the importance of a healthy microbiome. For example, double-blind trials have shown that people treated with lactobacillus and bifidobacterium (types of probiotics) experienced improvements in psychological distress, anxiety, and depression, and had decreased anger and hostility, less anxiety, and improved problem solving. Research has also shown that HPA-axis dysregulation can be reversed by treatment with lactobacillus and bifidobacterium. This research verifies the two-way communication between the digestive tract and the brain.

In addition, evidence shows that bowel disorders are often correlated with poor mood. In fact, 20% of patients with functional bowel disorders such as IBS have a diagnosable psychiatric illness. Almost one-third of patients with IBS have been found to have anxiety or depression.

Dysbiosis

Dysbiosis, an imbalance in gut bacteria, can result from anything that alters gut microbiota. The most common causes are antibiotics, oral contraceptives, hormone replacement therapy, acid-suppressing medications, corticosteroids, gastrointestinal infections, surgery, poor digestion, chronic constipation, chronic mental/emotional stress, a high sugar and refined carbohydrate diet, and food allergies. Dysbiosis can manifest in many ways, and may have a number of causes. The questionnaire below, adapted from the work of William Crook, MD, will help you determine what degree of dysbiosis you may have.

Dysbiosis Questionnaire

GENERAL HISTORY

10	Have you taken tetracyclines (e.g., Minocin) for acne for one month or longer?
10	Have you taken, or do you take, antibiotics for infections more than four times per year?
10	Have you taken birth control pills for more than two years?
5	Have you taken birth control pills for six months to two years?
10	Have you taken prednisone or other cortisone-like drugs (e.g., asthma medication)?
10	Does the smell of perfume, tobacco, or other odours or chemicals make you sick?
5	Do you crave sugars and breads?
_____	**Total score**

Symptoms

Enter **(1)** if symptom is mild; **(2)** if moderate or frequent; **(3)** if severe or constant

_____ Experience vaginal discharge or irritation

_____ Experience frequent bladder infections or incontinence

_____ Experience premenstrual syndrome or fluid retention

_____ Have difficulty getting pregnant

_____ Have frequent infections (sinus, lung, colds, etc.)

_____ Have allergies to foods or environmental substances

_____ Feel worse on rainy and snowy days, around molds or musty basements

_____ Experience feelings of anxiety and/or irritability

_____ Have insomnia

_____ Experience gas and bloating

_____ Experience constipation or diarrhea

_____ Have bad breath

_____ Have a difficult time concentrating (feel "spacey")

_____ Experience muscle weakness or painful joints

_____ Have nasal congestion

_____ Feel pressure behind or irritation of the eyes

_____ Have frequent headaches

_____ Generally "don't feel well" without an explanation or diagnosis

_____ Have thyroid problems

_____ Have muscle aches or weakness

_____ **Total score from all sections**

If you scored: Under 50 – You are considered to have mild dysbiosis. **50–90** – You are considered to have moderate dysbiosis. **90–120** – You are considered to have severe dysbiosis.

Bowel toxicity stress reduction tips

- If you suspect dysbiosis, take immediate steps to bring your intestinal flora back into balance by following these recommendations:
- Eat unprocessed foods – whole grains, beans, vegetables, fruit, nuts – high in natural fibre. Plant fibres found in natural foods absorb harmful compounds and encourage regular evacuation.
- Avoid antibiotics whenever possible; instead, seek safer, naturally immune-enhancing treatments for infections. Antibiotics kill beneficial bacteria in the colon, allowing yeast and other harmful organisms to flourish.
- Avoid simple sugars and other refined foods that stress the digestive and immune systems and encourage microbiota imbalance.
- Avoid hormone replacement therapy, birth control pills, and steroid medications such as cortisone whenever possible, and investigate natural alternatives. These drugs encourage yeast overgrowth since they increase blood sugar levels.
- Take steps to reduce the various stressors in your life. Unrelieved stress lowers immunity, enhancing the possibility of dysbiosis.

Dysbiosis treatment recommendations

The four components of the treatment for cleansing the bowel and decreasing the toxic overload are:

1. Make dietary changes to starve out candida and harmful bacteria.
2. Cleanse the bowel of harmful microflora and accumulated toxins.
3. Restore beneficial microflora.
4. Follow the moderate dysbiosis diet (see below).

The dysbiosis diet

The objective of the dysbiosis diet is to reduce the intake of foods that encourage the growth of harmful yeast and bacteria. Carefully follow this diet for a 10-week period.

Foods to avoid

- Sugars of all types, and foods that contain refined or simple sugars
- Dried fruit (e.g., raisins, prunes, dates)
- Fruit juices, both fresh and frozen

- Yeasted breads, pastries, and other baked goods (alternatives include corn tortillas and burritos, unyeasted crackers or rice cakes, sprouted breads, and yeast-free and sugar-free breads)
- Alcoholic beverages and malt products
- Peanuts and cashews
- Cow's milk (use in moderation on cereal or in coffee; alternatives include almond milk and goat's milk)
- Ice cream
- Antibiotics

Foods that can be eaten freely

- Fresh, unprocessed meats, poultry, and fish
- Eggs
- Raw nuts (except peanuts and cashews) and seeds
- Flaxseed and olive oil
- Low-carbohydrate vegetables such as all green leafy vegetables (chard, kale, celery, lettuce, spinach), broccoli, cabbage, and Brussels sprouts
- Butter and yogourt (in the absence of allergies to dairy products)

Foods that can be eaten cautiously

- Fruit (no more than two daily)
- Cereals and other whole grain products (ensure they are yeast free and sugar free)
- High-carbohydrate vegetables (e.g., squash, potatoes, carrots, beets)
- Cheese (small amounts, 2–3 times per week)

Monitor your intake of foods in the "eat with caution" category day by day. For example, if you have a high-carbohydrate vegetable for lunch (such as sweet potatoes), then have only a small serving of grains or pasta for dinner.

Additional treatment options

In addition to following the dysbiosis diet, it is very important to kill off unfriendly microbes, and to take a probiotic to restore the beneficial microflora. Various products decrease the load of toxic microbes, such as the following:

- Psyllium absorbs toxins and helps carry them out of the colon.

- Caprylic acid is a natural compound with antifungal properties that is effective in treating intestinal imbalances.

- Garlic supplements, grapefruit seed extract, peppermint oregano oil, and olive leaf extract all kill off unfriendly microbes.

- Psyllium seed is a bulking agent that helps eliminate toxins by encouraging regular bowel movements and by binding with stored waste products that normally are not eliminated.

- The herbs buckthorn *(Rhamnus cathartica, Rhamnus frangula)* and cascara sagrada *(Rhamnus purshiana)* encourage efficient bowel elimination, which is important for microbial balance. These herbs increase peristalsis (the muscular contractions of the bowel), thereby assisting with the removal of toxins.

Restoring Beneficial Microflora

Probiotics

The two most important friendly bacteria in our bodies are *Lactobacillus acidophilus* and *Bifidobacterium bifidum.* Lactobacilli and bifidobacteria in the intestines inhibit the growth of unfriendly organisms by producing antimicrobial factors. These bacteria are found in the fermented foods that most cultures use, such as yogourt, miso, tempeh, keifer, sauerkraut, and fermented juices. These foods, as well as probiotic supplements containing beneficial bacteria, benefit human health. A high-quality lactobacilli and bifidobacteria supplement will provide greater colonization of the friendly bacteria.

Daily use of probiotics while following the dysbiosis diet and cleansing protocols, and regular use thereafter, is recommended. If you eat foods that are high in friendly bacteria, then you do not need to take a daily supplement, though you may wish to use one at least two days a week to maintain adequate levels of the friendly microbes. The dysbiosis cleanse program should be considered as part of your general health and three brain health program once or twice a year to ensure a healthy gut-brain relationship. For those who experience irritable bowel syndrome a combination of *Bifidobacterium longum, Lactobacillus helveticus, Bacillus subtilis* and *Enterococcus faecium* have been proven effective. As a side benefit, addressing dysbiosis can help reduce stress and anxiety.

Exercise

Evidence suggests that exercise may increase the diversity of bacteria living in the gut. One study showed increased gut bacterial diversity and fewer markers of inflammation in athletes compared with controls. However, moderate exercise may be best; one study found that people who exercised anywhere from once a month to once a day had higher levels of brain-protecting BDNF than non-exercisers or extreme exercisers. Exercise has also been shown to have positive anti-inflammatory benefits, which may promote the health of the three brains.

Chronic Stress and the Adrenal Glands

"To understand the mechanism of stress gives physicians a new approach to treatment of illness, but it can also give us all a new way of life, a new philosophy to guide our actions in conformity with natural laws." – Hans Selye, MD

All individuals subjected to chronic and severe stress go through stages of adapting to these stressors. The stages of stress-induced damage were first studied by Canadian doctor Hans Selye. He gave us a greater understanding of how stress affects the entire body. If stress is prolonged, many people may develop adrenal insufficiency. The relationship between the stressors and the body's stress resistance determines when, and to what extent, ill health will result. Dr. Selye calls the body's mechanism for dealing with stress the general adaptation syndrome (GAS).

Adrenal Dysregulation

Adrenal dysregulation is one of the most prevalent conditions in our time, yet it is rarely diagnosed in Western medicine. Unfortunately, the milder forms of hypo- or hyperadrenia are missed or often misdiagnosed in health care practitioners' offices every day, even though all of the symptoms are present.

Although lab tests are a necessary part of a diagnosis, the narrow parameters often miss people in the earlier stages of a disease, called the preclinical range. At this stage, most people are told there is nothing wrong because the lab test is within the "normal" range. As a result, many people suffer unnecessarily for years. This is no surprise considering that lab tests are standardized according to statistical norms based on math instead of physiological optimal norms, which are based on signs and symptoms.

As you can see from Figure 2.2, the optimal functional range for the adrenals is very small, while the preclinical ranges for either hyper- or hypoadrenal functioning is the biggest piece of the bell curve. The extremes, Addison's disease and Cushing's syndrome, are diagnosable through conventional lab tests.

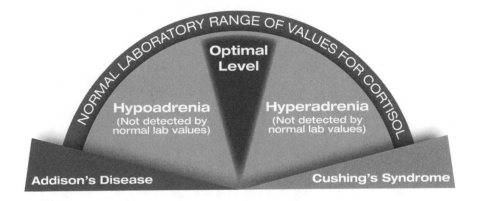

Figure 2.2 The range of values for cortisol

Adrenal fatigue symptoms for both hypo- and hyperfunction are very similar. They include:

- Fatigue/chronic fatigue
- Muscle weakness
- Anxiety, depression, mood swings
- Sleep disorders
- Irregular menses
- Hypoglycemia
- Inflammation
- Memory problems
- Difficulty losing weight
- Decreased immunity
- Low or high blood pressure
- Hair loss
- Low libido

Many people alternate between the two stages for years, some in a more hyper state and others more hypo. If left unchecked, these patients will eventually end up with severe adrenal exhaustion.

Table 2.1 provides a checklist to help you identify if you are showing symptoms of adrenal stress.

Table 2.1 Adrenal Stress Indicator

Write the number **1** beside symptoms you have had in the past; **2** beside symptoms that occur occasionally; **3** beside symptoms that occur often; **4** beside symptoms that occur frequently. Add up the total score.

_____ Blurred vision, spots in front of eyes

_____ Insomnia, frequent waking

_____ Hormonal imbalances (e.g., thyroid problems)

_____ History of asthma, bronchitis

_____ Prolonged exposure to stress (e.g., job, family, illness, caregiving)	_____ Air hunger (e.g., shortness of breath, yawning)
_____ Headaches	_____ Low back pain, knee problems, sore muscles
_____ Environmental or chemical exposure or sensitivities	_____ Excessive urination
_____ Hypoglycemia, blood sugar problems (e.g., mood swings)	_____ Excessive perspiration or no perspiration
_____ Food allergies	_____ Heart palpitations
_____ Poor concentration, memory problems (e.g., Alzheimer's)	_____ Edema of extremities or general edema
_____ Low energy, excessive fatigue	_____ Eyes light-sensitive
_____ Easily overwhelmed, inability to handle stress	_____ Cravings for sugar, salt, coffee, or other stimulants
_____ Post-exertion fatigue	_____ Alcohol intolerance
_____ Dizziness or fainting upon standing	_____ Recurrent colds or infections
_____ Inflammatory conditions (e.g., arthritis, bursitis)	_____ Digestive problems, ulcers
_____ Cold hands or feet	_____ Weight gain or weight loss
_____ Nervousness, anxiety, depression, irritability, anger	_____ High or low blood pressure
	_____ **Total score**

If you scored: 30–50: You have received an early-warning indicator that your adrenals are starting to weaken. **50–80:** Start with adrenal support. **80–100:** Your adrenals are taxed; you may want to add an adrenal glandular product. **Over 100:** You are suffering from adrenal exhaustion and will require long-term adrenal support.

Stress Support

Many disorders of the three brains, as well as most chronic diseases, have stress as one the main causes. As a result, most, if not all of us, would benefit from supporting the stress adaptive system, namely the adrenal glands.

Energy and Stress Support

Most people experience chronic stress of one form or another, and have or are beginning to experience symptoms of adrenal fatigue. It is therefore very important to support the stress response system.

Ashwagandha *(Withania somnifera)*

Ashwagandha is a well-researched adaptogen that has been shown to reduce levels of cortisol, which becomes elevated in stressful conditions. An animal study has shown that ashwagandha reduced brain levels of a marker of clinical anxiety comparable to the effects of lorazepam. Ashwagandha also exhibited an antidepressant effect comparable to that induced by imipramine. A patented *Withania somnifera* extract known as Sensoril has shown impressive clinical results in dealing with stress. It is standardized to contain the proper amounts of active ingredients that have been shown to promote anti-stress activity.

Dosage: 125 mg once or twice daily.

Asian ginseng *(Panax ginseng)*

Panax ginseng and ginsengs in general are adaptogens that have been shown to enhance the body's ability to cope with mental and physical stressors. Panax has been shown to be an effective treatment in chronic stress, improving mood, energy, intellectual performance, and a sense of well-being. Animal studies have shown that the stress-relieving and anti-anxiety effects were comparable to those of diazepam (Valium) but without the side effects (behavioural changes and sedative effects).

Dosage: depends on the standardization and dried herb equivalents. For a 4:1 extract standardized to contain 5–6% ginsenosides, 50 mg 2–4 times daily. For a dried extract, 200 mg 2–4 times daily.

Rhodiola *(Rhodiola rosea)*

Rhodiola has many proven benefits, including balancing stress hormones and thereby relieving symptoms of stress, preventing mental fatigue, improving mental focus and stamina, supporting cognitive function, and improving concentration.

Dosage: depends on the standardization and dried herb equivalents. For example a 10:1 extract means that 50 mg would provide 500 mg of the dried herb equivalent. Many herbs are standardized for the active ingredients. In rhodiola, the primary active ingredient is rosavin. Look for a product that is standardized to contain approximately 3.5% rosavin. Dosage for a 10:1 extract is 100–200 mg daily (1000–2000 dhe).

Choline

Choline deficiency may change the way the brain and adrenal glands respond to stress. Animal studies show impaired hormonal response to stress when choline is deficient in the diet. Choline supplementation increases acetylcholine synthesis and release in the brain, adrenal glands, muscles, and heart, all of which help counteract the many negative effects of mental and physical stress. Choline supports memory function, which can be compromised during chronic stress.

Dosage: depending on the source of choline, different doses are recommended.

Green Tea

Green tea contains potent antioxidants called catechins; epigallocatechin gallate (EGCG) is the most abundant catechin. Green tea also contains the amino acid L-theanine and caffeine, but unlike coffee, green tea helps keep people alert but calm. It has been shown to prevent oxidative stress, restore glutathione levels in the brain, and improve symptoms of chronic fatigue syndrome, a condition that is stress-induced.

Dosage: 300–600 mg daily, standardized to contain 60% catechins (40% EGCG).

 LOOK for a product such as...

Stress Less, that contains extracts of green tea, ashwagandha, rhodiola, and *Panax ginseng,* plus choline.

Calming Support

For those who feel wired and stressed during the day, it is important to support the nervous system to prevent the overproduction of stress hormones. The goal is to feel calm and centred rather than tired and wired during times of increased demands.

Relora

Relora is a proprietary blend that contains both magnolia *(Magnolia officinalis)* and phellodendron bark *(Phellodendron amurense).* Magnolia bark helps regulate the stress hormone cortisol and is helpful in reducing anxiety-related insomnia. Phellodendron is known for its anti-inflammatory and calming properties.

Dosage: 500–750 mg daily.

L-theanine

L-theanine's effects, for the most part, have to do with promoting relaxation. It has been shown to stimulate the brain's alpha waves, a state often related to meditation, suggesting that it has the ability to put users into a more relaxed mood. It also reduces beta waves, which are associated with hyperactivity, nervousness, and scattered mind chatter. Studies have shown that L-theanine reduces stress, helps with sleep, and increases mental alertness.

Dosage: 100–200 mg 1–3 times daily.

Magnesium

Magnesium is an important mineral for more than 300 biochemical reactions in the body. Deficiency can be caused by chronic stress.

Dosage: 400–800 mg daily.

Taurine

Taurine is an amino acid that acts as an inhibitory neurotransmitter. It suppresses the release of excitatory neurotransmitters like dopamine and norepinephrine, both of which are increased during stress.

Dosage: higher doses of 1000–5000 mg daily are often required for relaxation and anxiety.

General Stress Support

Probiotics and prebiotics

Animal studies indicate that the bacteria present in the gut in early life affect the development of the stress system and shape how the animal responds to stress in adulthood.

Bifidobacterium longum, a probiotic, has been shown to normalize anxiety in mice, while *Lactobacillus rhamnosus* has been shown to have a marked effect on gamma-aminobutyric acid (GABA) levels, lowering stress-induced cortisol levels and resulting in reduced anxiety and depressive behaviour. A study from Oxford University published in the *Journal of Psychopharmacology* in 2015 showed that people who took prebiotics had lower levels of cortisol in their saliva when they woke up in the morning, compared with people who took a placebo. Other studies show that a combination of *Bifidobacterium longum* and *Lactobacillus helveticus* have proven beneficial for stress related anxiety and depression.

Dosage: depends on the type of probiotic or combined probiotic/prebiotic. Follow the manufacturer's instructions.

Omega-3 essential fatty acids

The essential fatty acids eicosapentaenoic acid (EPA) and docosahexaenoic acid (DHA) have been shown to lower or blunt cortisol and epinephrine production during stress. Clinical studies have also shown that an imbalance in the dietary intake of fatty acids is linked to inflammation, impaired brain performance, and disease. When choosing an omega-3 product, try to make sure it is free from heavy metals such as lead and mercury, pesticides, and other contaminants. Look for a combined product that contains at least 1000 mg of EPA and DHA.

Dosage: for general health, 1000 mg daily; for inflammatory conditions, 3000 mg daily.

Vitamin C

Vitamin C is very important because it is used in the formation of adrenal hormones. During times of stress, the body's requirement for vitamin C can increase 10–20-fold.

Dosage: 2000–4000 mg daily (or until you begin to experience loose stools).

Vitamin B6

B6 is a necessary cofactor for the formation of several important neurotransmitters such as GABA, serotonin, and dopamine, which are commonly associated with stress.

Dosage: 100–250 mg daily.

Vitamin B12

B12 is thought to have an effect on helping to reset healthy secretion of cortisol during periods of stress, thus improving the stress response and quality of sleep.

Dosage: 1000–5000 mcg daily in the form of methylcobalamin.

Phosphatidylserine (PS)

PS can modulate the cortisol released in stressful situations. In a study of exercise-induced stress, cortisol was lower after exercise in healthy volunteers using PS versus a placebo. It is thought that PS affects the HPA response to stress. This may provide some insight into the effect of PS on depression, as elevated cortisol is a common finding in depression.

Dosage: 300 mg daily.

LOOK for a product such as...

Brilliant Mind, which contains PS and PC, green tea extract, and omega-3 fatty acids, to help prevent the overproduction of stress hormones and provide additional benefit to those who experience chronic stress.

Multivitamin

A multivitamin and mineral supplement will supply the essential nutrients that are cofactors for brain neurotransmitters and provide the B vitamins necessary to support the nervous system.

Dosage: depends on the type of product. Follow the suggested daily dosage from the manufacturer.

Meditation

Different types of meditation have been shown to result in psychological and biological changes that are associated with improved health. Meditation has been found to reduce blood pressure and heart rate, alter levels of melatonin and serotonin, suppress stress hormones, boost the immune system, promote positive mood states, reduce anxiety and pain, enhance self-esteem, and have a favourable influence on overall and spiritual quality of life in late-stage disease.

More than eight in ten North Americans think prayer or meditation can augment medical treatment, according to a survey released by the sponsor of Harvard Medical School's Spirituality and Healing in Medicine seminars. Just as we need physical exercise and good whole foods to keep our physical body healthy, we need daily spiritual exercises (contemplation, prayer, or meditation) to keep our minds and emotions balanced. Life is moving so quickly today that a meditative practice is more necessary than ever before.

Massage therapy

Studies have shown that massage therapy can decrease cortisol and increase serotonin and dopamine levels. The research reviewed studies on depression, pain syndrome, autoimmune conditions, immune disorders, stress on the job, stress of aging, and pregnancy stress. The results show that massage therapy led to an average decrease in cortisol of 31%, and average increases in the neurotransmitters serotonin and dopamine of 28% and 31% respectively.

Exercise

Everyone knows exercise can benefit overall health, but it also has direct stress-reducing benefits. Virtually any form of exercise can relieve stress. For example, exercise that gets the blood pumping, such as running, hiking, or racquetball, can increase the production of endorphins, the feel-good brain chemicals. As tensions and stress are released through exercise, sleep will improve, worries and anxieties will decrease, and you will feel more relaxed.

It doesn't take much; only two hours a week of moderate exercise or approximately an hour of vigorous exercise have been shown to provide anti-stress benefits. Choose an exercise you like to do. Any form of exercise of movement can help increase fitness and reduce stress, such as walking, climbing stairs, jogging, cycling, yoga, tai chi, gardening, swimming, or weight lifting, at least twice a week.

Exercise more, laugh more, listen to music more, meditate more, and spend more time in nature. There are many things you can do to help relieve stress. Most people know what makes them feel less stressed, so just do it!

Perception

Perception is what we think about a given situation, and it plays a very important role in our body's reaction to stress. The stress reaction is the result of many complex interacting factors, such as the influence of the actual stressor as well as our perception of the stressor. How we perceive the event is part of what determines whether or not the fight-or-flight response is triggered. For example, if our perception is influenced by a negative and pessimistic attitude, then the stressor will be perceived as more of a threat than it would be if we had a more optimistic and positive outlook.

So, can changing how you perceive stress make you healthier? The answer is "Yes". A 2012 study used data from a stress questionnaire that tracked over 28,000 adults. The first question was about how much stress they experienced, and the next question was if they felt that their stress was harmful to their health. Over the next eight years, researchers tracked public death records of the participants to see who among them had died. The results showed that worrying and believing that stress was harmful to their health predicted an early death. Shockingly, those who were under high levels of stress, but who did not believe that it caused them harm, had much better health and longevity. They even had a lower risk of dying compared to those who had less stress, but who held the belief that their stress was harmful.

"The greatest weapon against stress is our ability to choose one thought over another."
– William James

Once we fully understand that we have choices in our lives, we come to realize that the majority of the limitations placed upon us are those we create with our own belief systems and ideologies. If our thought formations help create our reality, we can use and manipulate them to contribute to the creation of good health (or conversely, of disease). Listen carefully to your spoken and unspoken thoughts and observe where they are leading you. As evidence has shown, in many cases you are your own master.

The attitude of gratitude: remember to say thank you!

New research conducted by Robert A. Emmons, PhD, of the University of California, and Michael E. McCullough, of the University of Miami, shows that the "attitude of gratitude" has been linked to better health, sounder sleep, less anxiety and depression, higher long-term satisfaction with life, and kinder behaviour toward others. In the study, people kept a brief "gratitude journal" – just one sentence for each of five things that they were grateful for, done once a week. There were significant effects after only two months. Compared with a control group, the people keeping the gratitude journal were more optimistic and felt happier. They reported fewer physical problems and spent more time working out.

"If you want to sleep more soundly, count blessings, not sheep", Dr. Emmons advises in *Thanks!,* his book on gratitude research.

For more information on stress, refer to *Stress and the Disease Connection: A Complete Guide,* by Karen Jensen, ND and Marita Schauch, ND, and *Stress, Anxiety and Insomnia: What the Drug Companies Won't Tell You and Your Doctor Doesn't Know,* by Michael T. Murray, ND.

Brain Busters

Genetics, social environment, and nutrition all play vital roles in brain development and function. However, a number of other factors can also negatively affect the three brains. This chapter reviews two of the most common brain busters: inflammation, and food allergies and intolerances. Understanding how these factors affect the head brain and, for many conditions, all three brains, can provide information on how to treat and even prevent many common brain disorders.

The Brain Aflame

Inflammation is the first response of the immune system to infection, injury, or irritation from a foreign substance. The purpose of the inflammatory response is to remove debris, attack foreign invaders, remove cellular waste, and encourage the healing process.

Inflammation of the brain is a protective reaction that aids in the repair and regeneration of damaged brain cells. If it continues for too long, however, inflammation does more harm than good, damaging neurons and contributing to brain disorders such as depression, bipolar and other mood disorders, traumatic brain injury, Alzheimer's disease, Parkinson's disease, and fatigue. Figure 3.1 shows the effects of chronic inflammation on the brain.

Chronic inflammation causes oxidative stress: an imbalance between the overproduction of free radicals (unstable atoms or groups of atoms) and the ability of antioxidants to protect the cells. Free radicals damage cells by reacting with proteins and cell membrane fatty acids, permanently impairing their function. The brain is approximately 60% fat, so damage from free radicals can be significant.

Inflammation also has a profound effect on the heart brain. For example, Danish researchers found that elevated levels of a C-reactive protein, which the body produces in response to inflammation, are associated with an increased risk for psychological distress and depression in the general population. In addition, elevated C-reactive protein is commonly found in people with cardiovascular disease, in particular atherosclerosis.

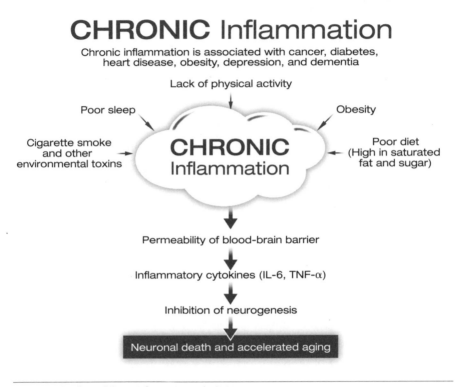

Figure 3.1 The Effects of Chronic Inflammation on the Brain

Some causes of brain inflammation include increased oxidative stress, disturbed immune function, food allergens, imbalance in gut microbiota (leaky gut), psychological stressors, and other stressors such as environmental toxins, heavy metals, pesticides, electromagnetic frequencies (EMFs), and infections (virus, bacteria, or moulds).

Prevention and Treatment of Inflammation

Drugs are available for chronic inflammation, such as aspirin and other over-the-counter non-steroidal anti-inflammatory drugs (NSAIDs), but there are also many natural ways to prevent and treat inflammation. For example, an anti-inflammatory diet, such as the Mediterranean diet (which consists of foods containing omega-3 fatty acids such as fish, walnuts, and flaxseed oil), can help prevent inflammation. Probiotics are also helpful because the gut is home to nearly 70% of the immune system. As a result, foods that support healthy gut microbiota, such as sauerkraut, miso, kimchi, kefir, and yogourt, can also be added to the diet. (Refer to Chapter 7 for more information on anti-inflammatory supplement support for mood disorders and Chapter 9 for support for cognitive disorders.)

Curcumin *(Curcuma longa)*

Curcumin is the most active compound in turmeric, commonly used in curry. It has potent anti-inflammatory, antioxidant, and lipophilic, as well as metal chelation effects. Research has shown that curcumin is comparable to common prescription medications like hydrocortisone and over-the-counter medications such as ibuprofen in the treatment of inflammation. It has proven to be effective in the treatment of dementias, including Alzheimer's, as well as other brain disorders such as depression and symptoms related to traumatic brain injury. Curcumin is able to enter the brain, bind, and destroy the beta-amyloid plaques present in Alzheimer's, with reduced toxicity. However, curcumin is difficult for the body to absorb, and even very high doses have failed to increase blood levels. Formulations specifically designed to increase absorption more effectively raise blood and tissue levels and provide better results. Reducing the particle size is the best way to optimize absorption and bioavailability.

Dosage: 300 mg daily.

Boswellia *(Boswellia serrata)*

Boswellia, also known as Indian frankincense, contains boswellic acids and has been used as a major anti-inflammatory agent for centuries. Many studies have shown that boswellia is just as effective as NSAIDs, which are the most commonly used treatment for inflammation. Boswellia reduces post-injury inflammation and improves neurobehavioural and cognitive dysfunction that result from traumatic brain injury, which is a common cause of dementia.

Dosage: 300–500 mg daily of an extract standardized to contain 30–40% boswellic acids.

Omega-3 essential fatty acids

Essential fatty acids (EFAs) are as effective as NSAIDs for reducing inflammatory pain, and they are a much safer alternative. Clinical studies show that an imbalance in the dietary intake of fatty acids is linked to impaired brain performance and disease. When choosing an omega-3 product, ensure it is free from heavy metals such as lead and mercury, pesticides, and other contaminants. Look for a combined product that contains at least 1000 mg of eicosapentaneoic acid (EPA) and docosahexaenonic acid (DHA). (See Chapter 6 for more information on EFAs.)

Dosage: 1000 mg daily for general health; 3000 mg daily for inflammatory conditions.

Food Allergies and Brain Disorders

Allergies are disorders of the immune system that are caused by an improper immune response. Since food is something that we consume on a day-to-day basis, it is easy to appreciate why food represents one of the largest challenges that the immune system has to deal with. Certain food allergens or inhaled particles, such as dust or pollen, can trigger a defence mechanism. The immune system releases antibodies, causing a wide variety of symptoms, including brain disorders. The two commonly-produced antibodies are IgG and IgE. IgG reactions occur over several hours or days, whereas IgE reactions occur within minutes or hours of exposure. About 75% of the antibodies we produce are IgGs.

The digestive system is a very important component when dealing with allergies. A large portion (70%) of our immune system resides in our gut, referred to as gut-associated lymph tissue (GALT). When certain foods react with GALT repeatedly over time, inflammation causes the gut brain to become leaky. Poorly digested foods and allergens are able to cross the leaky membrane and move into the blood stream, causing stress on the immune system. (See Chapter 2 for more information on leaky gut.)

Allergy Versus Food Sensitivity/Intolerance

Food intolerance, also known as non-IgE-mediated food hypersensitivity or non-allergic food hypersensitivity, refers to difficulty in digesting certain foods. It is important to note that food intolerance is different from food allergy. Food allergy triggers the immune system, while food intolerance does not. An allergen is a protein that causes a food allergy. Food intolerance is usually due to an enzyme deficiency, meaning that a substance in the food is not digested properly. Food intolerance reactions can be severe and extremely unpleasant, but are rarely life-threatening. However, in some cases of food allergy, there can be a severe and life-threatening allergic reaction (anaphylaxis) to certain foods.

As those with food allergies know, food sensitivities and allergies can have a profound effect on the head brain and cognitive function as well as the gut brain. Head brain cells are not alone in being able to communicate through the action of neurotransmitters. Immune cells in the digestive tract, blood, and other body tissues also have receptors to many neurotransmitters. One study looked at the connection between allergies and schizophrenia and autism, and found that among autistic children, 87% had higher levels of IgG antibodies to gluten and 90% had higher levels of these antibodies to casein, the protein found in milk and milk products. Figures were similar for people with schizophrenia.

I had been in practice as a naturopathic doctor for almost 20 years when parents brought their eight-year-old son to see me. They had tried everything they knew of to help him and didn't know what to do. The mother told me that "he came out of the womb aggressive, angry, and destructive", and at eight years old he was rapidly heading toward a life in juvenile detention centres.

I was shocked when I heard their story, as I had never seen such dramatic aggressive behaviour in a young child. I was overwhelmed and frankly didn't know where to start in providing some help for this devastated family. So I simply recommended the basics. I asked them to remove sugar and refined products, dairy products, and all wheat products from the child's diet. The only supplement I gave the child was probiotics.

When they returned for a follow-up visit six weeks later, I couldn't believe what they told me. The mother said, "We have never met this child before; it is like meeting him for the first time". His behaviour had changed completely; he was no longer aggressive or angry and got along with other children and his parents. Only when he inadvertently ate a food he should not have did he turn into a "monster", in the mother's words. These small changes in diet resulted in significant changes in the family's life.

Other conditions caused by allergies or sensitivities include anxiety, depression, insomnia, and attention deficit/ hyperactivity disorder (ADD/ADHD). Symptoms of head brain allergies include brain fog, poor concentration, cognition problems, moodiness, sudden mood changes, crying, vulgarity, becoming withdrawn, irritability, and anger. Symptoms of gut brain allergies include vomiting, reflux, abdominal pain, and diarrhea or constipation.

Allergy testing

Conventionally accepted medical approaches for allergy assessment include skin scratch tests in which small punctures are made on the skin with needles containing tiny amounts of allergens. This test is limited because it only tests IgE (immediate) reactions. A blood test called enzyme-linked immunosorbent assay (ELISA) is used to test both IgE and IgG reactions, providing a more comprehensive analysis to determine both immediate and delayed food and environmental allergies.

Gluten Intolerance and Brain Drain

Evidence of neurological symptoms in patients with established celiac disease has been reported since 1966. However, it was not until 30 years later that gluten sensitivity was first shown to lead to neurological dysfunction. Gluten sensitivity, also referred to as non-celiac gluten sensitivity (NCGS), may be even more of a cause of psychiatric illness than overt celiac disease. Gluten sensitivity occurs at six times the rate of celiac disease. Gluten intolerance causes inflammation throughout the body and profoundly affects all three brains.

Gluten intolerance is a growing problem worldwide, but especially in North America and Europe. Gluten is relatively new to our diet; humans did not frequently consume it over the last two million years. When we eat a diet high in foods that contain gluten, it causes inflammation which, as we discussed, is the cornerstone of most chronic disease. Several studies have suggested a relationship between NCGS and brain disorders, including autism, schizophrenia, Alzheimer's, anxiety, depression, and ADHD.

Many experts estimate that 1 in 100 people have celiac disease, and this number does not include those with undiagnosed celiac disease. Only 1 in 4,700 who suffer from celiac disease have actually been diagnosed; the number is even higher when undiagnosed cases of NCGS are included. The estimated number of people suffering from gluten problems is closer to 1 in 30.

Researchers at the University of Maryland School of Medicine have found that the protein zonulin regulates the permeability of the intestine. Zonulin proteins are found within intestinal cells and their production is triggered by various foreign bacteria. Zonulin in normal amounts acts as a gatekeeper, opening the spaces between cells, allowing some substances to pass through while keeping harmful bacteria and toxins out. Elevated levels of zonulin, due to leaky gut and gluten ingestion, cause inflammation. As in the gut, zonulin is also involved in the regulation of the impenetrable barrier between the blood stream and the brain, known as the blood-brain barrier (BBB).

*Grains that **contain gluten** include barley, bulgur, couscous, graham flour, kamut, matzo, rye, durum semolina, spelt, triticale, wheat, and wheat germ.*

*The following grains are **gluten-free:** amaranth, arrowroot, buckwheat, corn, millet, quinoa, rice, sorghum, soy, tapioca, and potato flour.*

The wheat protein gliadin mimics the effects of foreign bacteria, and it also triggers elevated levels of zonulin. Gliadin is a complex of proteins found within what is referred to as gluten. The term is misleading because gluten is not one molecule. Rather, gluten is made up of two main groups of proteins: glutenins and gliadins. Gliadin is considered the primary class of proteins in wheat that cause allergy or intolerance. Wheat proteins stimulate antibodies that cross-react with neurological structures, which may explain how they contribute to neurological damage, neuropathy, schizophrenia, autism, seizures, and behavioural disorders.

If you are even vaguely suspicious of gluten sensitivity, try following a special diet for a trial period. Weeks or months may be required before a marked improvement appears after wheat, rye, barley, and oats, are removed from the diet. Re-introduction of these grains into the diet usually produces a relapse in months, days, or even hours if you are sensitive to these foods. If this occurs, it is important to strictly adhere to the diet and to be aware of the exact ingredients of the food. By eliminating the offending foods, irritability, mood swings, compulsive behaviour, and many other psychiatric disorders will improve if they are caused by these foods.

PERSONAL EXPERIENCE WITH WHEAT INTOLERANCE

My life changed when I was 40 years old. Until then I had suffered from irritable bowel problems and regular periods of debilitating brain fog. For no reason, or so it seemed, my brain would just shut down, my eyes would glaze over, and I would be unable to articulate what my scrambled brain was trying to convey. When I was younger, my parents took me to various doctors and I had the standard allergy tests. Everything appeared to be normal. It wasn't until my second year of naturopathic college at age 40, when my instructor used me to demonstrate a technique for testing for food intolerances, that I found the cause of these debilitating symptoms. It was determined that I was sensitive to wheat, spelt, durum, kamut – basically the entire wheat family. I was also informed that I had dysbiosis.

I was skeptical, but I decided that I had nothing to lose by eliminating wheat from my diet and following a dysbiosis protocol for two months. It felt like a miracle. The clouds cleared from my brain, my bloated abdomen disappeared, my bowel movements normalized, and I didn't feel like I was mentally slow; it was the beginning of a new chapter with a new level of well-being. Even today, 30 years later, I have to avoid any and all foods that contain wheat. It is so much easier today than it was 30 years ago, as gluten-free foods are readily available due to the increasing number of people who are avoiding gluten, either by choice or by necessity.

Dairy Products

Dairy allergies or intolerances cause different reactions in the body and head and gut brains. The most common reactions include digestive problems, skin issues, sinusitis, and excess mucus. Autism, schizophrenia, depression, and mood disorders have also been linked to dairy allergy.

While it is not well known, there are genetically different cows: A1 cows and A2 cows. All cows used to be A2 cows until a naturally occurring genetic mutation in European cows changed the genetics of milk-producing cow herds. The main proteins in milk are whey and casein. Casein is the most abundant overall, and the genetic variations of A1 and A2 refer to a specific type of casein. Populations that consume milk containing high levels of casein A2 variant have a lower incidence of cardiovascular disease and type 1 diabetes. Consumption of A2 milk may also be associated with less severe symptoms of autism and schizophrenia. In addition, the beta-caseins from breast milk help the newborn immune and gastrointestinal systems develop properly.

However, the casein in A1 milk has been shown in animal studies to cause inflammation in the small intestines, along with changes in endocrine (hormone), nervous, and immune systems. A1 milk also causes brain fog, sleep problems, and poor concentration, and has been linked to more serious neurological disorders such as schizophrenia and autism.

Goat's milk, as well as sheep and buffalo milk, contains A2 beta-casein. Raw milk, while often from cows, is typically produced from small herds of Jersey and Guernsey cows, both of which contain a high percentage of A2 beta-casein. Most dairies use mainly Holstein cows, which produce a majority of A1 beta-casein.

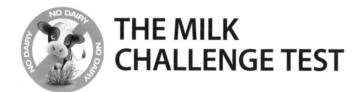

THE MILK CHALLENGE TEST

- For the first six weeks, avoid all dairy products, including butter.

- If symptoms improve, then introduce A2 milk products for 2–3 weeks. If your symptoms do not return, then you may be sensitive to A1 milk and you can continue with A2 sources such as goat or sheep milk products. Most people who can tolerate A2 milk also tolerate butter, even if from A1 cows, because it is primarily fat and has little casein.

- If your symptoms return even on A2 milk products, then avoid both A1 and A2 dairy products and switch to alternative milks such as almond, hemp, or rice.

- If your symptoms do not improve when all milk products are eliminated for six weeks, then they may not be due to a milk issue. You may need to try eliminating other foods or start working with a naturopathic doctor or alternative health care practitioner to determine the source of your allergy.

Sugar

Sugar suppresses the activity of a key growth hormone in the brain called brain-derived neurotrophic factor (BDNF). This hormone promotes the health and maintenance of neurons in the brain. It plays a vital role in memory and learning by triggering the growth of new connections between neurons. BDNF levels are critically low in people with depression and schizophrenia, which explains why both syndromes often lead to shrinkage of key brain regions over time. The microbiota also influences brain chemistry and behaviour directly. Intestinal dysbiosis alters BDNF and contributes to mental health disorders. Sugar consumption promotes inflammation and is a main cause of microbiota imbalance, which affects the three brains.

A recent cross-cultural study published in the *British Journal of Psychiatry* linked refined sugar consumption to mental illness. Clinical studies have linked sugar to depression, anxiety, suicide, irritability, anger outbursts, fatigue, and lethargy. Although sugar may not be categorized as a brain allergy or sensitivity, it is a mood-altering drug.

Researchers at Princeton University studying binging and dependency found that when animals ingested large amounts of sugar, their brains underwent changes similar to the changes in the brains of people who abuse illegal drugs like cocaine and heroin. The animals that drank large amounts of sugar water when hungry experienced behavioural changes, signs of withdrawal, and even long-lasting effects that resembled cravings.

The high consumption of sugar primarily linked to the standard North American diet is a problem of great magnitude. The prevalence of sugar addiction may largely explain the exponential increases in mental and physical illness in recent decades. Despite medical advances, chronic illness has been on the rise; one report indicated that chronic illness in children has quadrupled in a generation. The ever-increasing consumption of sugar and prevalence of environmental toxic stressors run parallel to that of the increase in mental and physical illness.

For general health and brain health, try to eliminate sugars and all refined simple starches (anything white such as bread, pasta, crackers, and pastry) for a couple of weeks to see if there is a change in energy, mental clarity, moods, aches, or digestion and elimination. If there is a favourable response, consider making this a permanent change in your diet.

More Brain Busters

In addition to inflammation and food allergies and intolerances, which were discussed in Chapter 3, a number of other factors can negatively affect brain function. These include hypertension and coronary artery disease, metabolism, mental health disorders and methylation disorders, thyroid disorders, and a range of toxins. Several tests are available that can help identify possible risk factors and allow for early intervention and treatment.

The Influence of the Heart Brain on the Head Brain

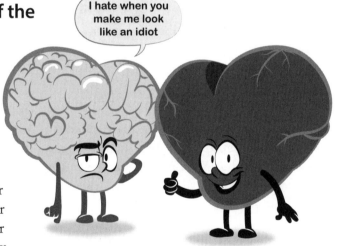

Hypertension and Coronary Artery Disease

Normal blood pressure is when the top number (systolic) is 120 or lower and the bottom number (diastolic) is 80 or below. Prehypertensive blood pressure is indicated by a top number between 120 and 139 and a bottom number between 80 and 89. Blood pressure greater than 140 over 90 is considered high.

Uncontrolled high blood pressure damages the brain's structure and function in individuals as young as 40. In a study published in the *Lancet Neurology* in December 2012, people with hypertension and prehypertension showed accelerated brain aging, damage to white matter, and reduced volume of grey matter in the brain. The increased risk of brain injury and atrophy leads to reduced cognitive ability and a greater chance of dementia. Hypertension is also thought to be directly associated with vascular dementia, and preliminary evidence suggests an association between elevated blood pressure and impairments in cognitive functioning.

The risk of elevated blood pressure among children and adolescents rose 27% during a 13-year period, according to research published in the *American Heart Association's Journal of Hypertension* in July 2013. There is evidence that childhood hypertension can lead to adult hypertension, and it is a known risk factor for coronary artery disease (CAD). The presence of childhood hypertension may contribute to the early development of CAD.

The neurological effects of hypertension in children are under-recognized. These children and adolescents are more likely to have learning disabilities and deficiencies in executive function that may be due to abnormal regulation of cerebral blood flow.

Higher body mass, larger waistlines, obesity, poor diet, and lack of exercise may be the reasons for elevated blood pressure. The good news is that these risk factors are mainly treatable and preventable through diet and lifestyle changes.

New evidence suggests a strong link between dementias and heart disease and is also finding many similarities between the two diseases. (Refer to Chapter 9 for more information.)

Metabolism and the Brain

The connection between metabolic disturbances and psychiatric disorders has been strengthened by ongoing human clinical studies. The results indicate numerous and complex interactions between metabolism and the brain leading to depression, anxiety disorders, dementias, and inflammation of the heart and gut brains.

The Role of Insulin and the Three Brains

The brain is only 2% of the body's mass, but approximately 25% of total body glucose is required for proper brain function, reflecting the high metabolic demand of neural processing. The brain is a particularly energy-intensive organ, and despite this high need for glucose, it has traditionally been viewed as functioning independently of insulin. However, this view has recently been challenged. Researchers have identified insulin receptors, insulin, and insulin-sensitive glucose transporters on both neurons and support cells throughout the brain and spinal cord, suggesting that insulin is required for normal cognitive and emotional functions. Insulin dysregulation also appears to be an important factor in the development of several psychiatric disorders. Proceedings of the

National Academy of Sciences in March 2015 reported that insulin resistance in the brain causes anxiety and depressive-like behaviours.

An intimate link exists between the brain and the metabolism of sugar, one that has been too long overlooked by the fields of neuroscience and psychiatry. The primary cause of the poor insulin receptor response is the chronic over-production of insulin due to stress and/or a diet high in sugar and refined carbohydrate foods or food with a high glycemic index (GI). The GI measures how quickly blood sugar increases after eating a particular food. The higher the GI, the faster the rise and fall of blood sugar. (Refer to Chapter 5 for more information on the GI.)

The gut microbiota has been identified as a contributor to metabolic diseases. It has been shown that obese individuals have different proportions of gut bacteria compared with lean individuals. This microbial imbalance seems to interfere with intestinal permeability, which can lead to impairment of insulin signalling. Recently, research has pointed out that the gut microbiome could be an important contributor to the development of type 2 diabetes.

The links between insulin resistance and the heart brain and the associated dyslipidemia, hypertension, hypercoagulability, and atherosclerosis are numerous and complex.

Mental Health Disorders and Methylation Disorders

Methylation is one of the body's most important and common chemical processes. It occurs in every cell of the body, and is essential for a wide range of critical functions in the body. Abnormal methylation has been shown to trigger brain inflammation, Alzheimer's disease, autism, and autoimmune diseases, to name a few.

The early work of Dr. Abram Hoffer paved the way in this area, providing an essential framework for the role of nutrients in brain biochemistry. Nutrients are the primary building blocks for all biochemical activity, including neurotransmitter synthesis. Dr. Carl Pfeiffer was an early pioneer in the research of how methylation problems lead to many different mental health and degenerative brain disorders. He discovered that by supplying the missing nutrients in the methylation process, many of these mental health problems were effectively treated. William Walsh, PhD, expanding on the earlier work of doctors Pfeiffer and Hoffer, has launched the biochemistry of mental illness into new arenas, thanks in part to recent discoveries and advances in genetics and epigenetics.

Thyroid Disorders and the Three Brains

Recent studies indicate that one in three Canadians has a thyroid disorder and of those, as many as 50% are undiagnosed. The psychological symptoms that commonly accompany hyperthyroidism (overactive) and hypothyroidism (underactive), the two most common thyroid disorders, can be easily mistaken for mental health problems.

The Role of the Thyroid Gland

The thyroid's job is to increase the body's metabolic rate by increasing the activity of the mitochondria (the body's energy producers). The mitochondria use oxygen to convert energy from food into carbon dioxide, water, heat, and energy for the body. Thyroid hormones are responsible for maintaining body temperature, stimulating protein synthesis, increasing the use of glucose, and breaking down fats for energy production. They speed up the elimination of cholesterol into bile from the liver. Thyroid hormones also affect mood, emotions, memory, and the way we think by increasing the growth of nervous tissue.

Hypothyroidism

Hypothyroidism (underactive or low thyroid function) occurs when the thyroid gland fails to produce sufficient amounts of the thyroid hormones thyroxine (T4) and triiodothyronine (T3), or if there is a failure in the conversion of T4 to T3. It is more common in females, affecting 20–25% of the female population in North America, while only about 10% of the male population experience hypothyroidism.

Since hypothyroidism usually develops slowly, and the early complaints are often vague, the diagnosis is often overlooked. However, the physical changes that accompany the illness are characteristic: dry, rough skin; pale and puffy complexion; loss of hair; change in voice; decreased appetite; etc. Psychological disturbances are often the main complaints that bring hypothyroid patients to the health care practitioner.

Mental emotional symptoms of hypothyroidism include:

- Progressive loss of interest and initiative
- Slowing of mental processes
- Poor memory for recent events
- Flatness of the personality
- Intellectual deterioration
- Depression
- Muddled thinking, brain fog

Hypothyroidism is much more common than hyperthyroidism.

Hyperthyroidism

Hyperthyroidism is a condition whereby the thyroid produces increased levels of the thyroid hormones T4 and T3. Graves' disease, which is another autoimmune disease, accounts for up to 85% of all cases of hyperthyroidism. Psychological disturbances are quite common with thyroid hyperactivity and can be part of the early picture.

Mental and emotional symptoms of hyperthyroidism include:

- Marked anxiety and tension
- Emotional volatility
- Impatience and irritability
- Lack of focus and attention
- Exaggerated sensitivity to noise
- Depression and sadness
- Sleep problems
- Changes in appetite

Chapter 2 discussed the effect of stress and stress hormones, particularly cortisol, on the three brains. Another of cortisol's important functions is to act in concert with thyroid hormones, making the thyroid work more efficiently. Cortisol is very important for normal thyroid function, and this is why many people who have an imbalance in adrenal cortisol levels usually have thyroid symptoms. Every cell in the body has receptors for both cortisol and thyroid, and nearly every cellular process requires optimal functioning of the thyroid.

Thyroid Disorders and the Head Brain

Many people who have thyroid disorders are wrongly diagnosed and treated with medications for a mental health problem, or in extreme cases, hospitalized for mental illness. In chronic untreated cases of hypothyroidism, many people, especially the elderly, may appear demented, confused, and have memory loss; these symptoms are often misdiagnosed as dementia or Alzheimer's. Research has also shown that even preclinical hypothyroidism is associated with memory impairment. In the treatment of depression not related to any diagnosed thyroid imbalance, the addition of L-thyroxine (medication for hypothyroidism) augments the effects of antidepressant drugs.

Thyroid Disorders and the Gut Brain

Hippocrates said "All disease begins in the gut". Today, we are just beginning to understand how right he was. Poor gut health can suppress thyroid function and trigger Hashimoto's disease, an autoimmune thyroid disorder. Low thyroid function can also lead to an inflamed and leaky gut, as illustrated in Figure 4.1.

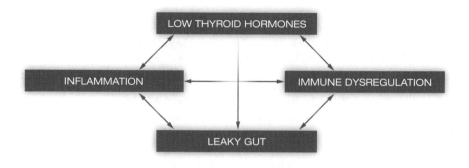

Figure 4.1 Hypothyroidism and "leaky gut"

- The thyroid influences the gut brain in several ways, including:

- When the intestinal barrier becomes permeable, called leaky gut, large protein molecules escape into the bloodstream triggering an immune response. The immune response plays a role in the development of auto-immune diseases such as Hashimoto's thyroiditis.

- Thyroid hormones strongly influence the tight junctions that form the gut barrier that protects the gut mucosal lining from stress-induced cellular damage. During examination of people with gastric ulcers, researchers found low T3 and T4, and abnormal levels of reverse T3.

- One very important role of the gut bacteria is to assist in converting T4 into the active form of thyroid hormone, T3. This conversion requires healthy gut bacteria. Intestinal dysbiosis, discussed in Chapter 2, significantly reduces the conversion of T4 to T3.

- Inflammation is commonly caused by stress-induced elevated cortisol, which decreases T3.

- Hypochlorhydria, or low stomach acid, also increases intestinal permeability, causing inflammation and microbiota imbalances.

Thyroid Disorders and the Heart Brain

The cardiovascular signs and symptoms of thyroid disease are some of the most profound and clinically relevant findings that accompany both hyperthyroidism and hypothyroidism. Scientists have identified a previously unknown group of nerve cells that develop in the brain with the aid of thyroid hormone, which is produced in the thyroid gland. Individuals who produce too much or too little thyroid hormone risk developing problems with these nerve cells. This, in turn, has an effect on the function of the heart, leading to cardiovascular disease.

It is well known that patients with untreated hyperthyroidism or hypothyroidism often develop heart problems as a result of thyroid hormone affecting the heart directly. However, this new research shows that thyroid hormone also affects the heart indirectly, through the newly discovered neurons in the head brain.

Hypothyroidism and the heart brain

The most common cardiovascular signs and symptoms of hypothyroidism may include blood pressure changes, alterations in lipid metabolism, decreased cardiac contractility, decreased cardiac output, accelerated atherosclerosis and coronary artery disease, and increased stroke risk.

Although subclinical hypothyroidism is often considered to be asymptomatic, many people have symptoms in the early stages of thyroid hormone deficiency. Lipid metabolism is altered and cholesterol levels appear to rise in parallel with thyroid-stimulating hormone (TSH) in hypothyroidism. C-reactive protein, a risk factor for heart disease, is also commonly increased in subclinical hypothyroidism. In addition, atherosclerosis, coronary heart disease, and myocardial infarction risk are increased in women with subclinical hypothyroidism. (Refer to the section on thyroid testing below for more information on lab values to determine optimal thyroid function.)

Hyperthyroidism and the heart brain

Hyperthyroidism and thyrotoxicosis, conditions that result from excess thyroid hormone, are associated with palpitations, tachycardia, exercise intolerance, shortness of breath on exertion, and sometimes atrial fibrillation. Cardiac contractility is enhanced, and resting heart rate and cardiac output are increased.

Subclinical hyperthyroidism is characterized by a low or undetectable serum TSH concentration in the presence of normal levels of serum T4 and T3. There may be no clinical signs or symptoms, however studies show that individuals are at risk for many of the cardiovascular manifestations associated with overt hyperthyroidism. The prevalence of subclinical hyperthyroidism appears to increase with advancing age. In a 10-year cohort study of older patients, a low TSH was associated with increased risk for cardiovascular mortality and atrial fibrillation.

Primary pulmonary hypertension is a progressive disease that leads to right heart failure and premature death, and is often of unknown origin. Recently, a link to thyroid disease has been identified. In one study of 40 patients with primary pulmonary hypertension, more than 22% of patients were determined to have hypothyroidism. Some evidence exists that autoimmune disease may play a role in both hypothyroid- and hyperthyroid-linked cases of primary pulmonary hypertension. Thyroid disease should be considered in the differential diagnosis of primary pulmonary hypertension.

Testing and Diagnosis

The hormones produced by the thyroid, T4 and T3, regulate the body's metabolism by controlling body temperature, the synthesis of protein, and the release of energy from the cells. T4 is the most abundant thyroid hormone produced (about 93%), and at one time was thought to be the active hormone. However, we now know that T3 is 3–5 times more biologically active, and that it is the active hormone in target cells. Most of T4 is converted to T3 in the liver, kidneys, and body cells (about 80%), and the thyroid is responsible for the rest.

TSH is secreted by the pituitary and stimulates the production of thyroid hormones. If the level of T4 and T3 hormones falls too low, more TSH is secreted; if the level is too high, less TSH is secreted. Lab test results may seem counterintuitive, but the higher the level of TSH, the lower the functioning of the thyroid.

Commonly, TSH is the only blood test ordered by most medical doctors, and thyroid function is considered "normal" if TSH falls between 0.38 and 5.5 IU/mL. The current lab tests in Canada indicate that a person has preclinical hypothyroidism if TSH is greater than 3.0 IU/mL but less than 5.5 IU/mL, but even at this point most health care practitioners do not consider treatment. Preclinical or suboptimal levels refer to results that fall in the normal range, yet the person has the classic symptoms of hypothyroidism.

However, naturopathic doctors and some medical doctors are now using a new "norm" for interpreting TSH results, and treat for hypothyroidism if TSH is above 1.9 IU/mL, especially if accompanied by low thyroid symptoms. Although most health care practitioners will only test TSH, it is important to measure the actual T4 and T3 levels to get a more accurate picture of the function of the thyroid. Remember that because T4 must be converted to the active T3 form, tests that only measure T4 don't illustrate the whole thyroid picture. It is possible that although circulating T4 levels are in a healthy range, there might be a problem converting T4 to T3.

Be sure to ask your health care practitioner to test levels of both hormones. TSH alone and the old lab reference range are often inadequate, and many hypothyroid patients suffer needlessly for years. It is particularly important to test for thyroid disorders in the aging if there are signs related to dementia such as memory loss, confusion, and general apathy.

Hypothyroidism is often more prevalent in older women, and for this reason older women should be regularly screened for low thyroid during routine annual physical examinations. It is also important to test men for thyroid disorders, especially those who have been under chronic stress or who are aging. Thyroid problems are often not taken into consideration by health care practitioners, even when men exhibit most of the classic signs of hypothyroidism.

Toxins in the Three Brains

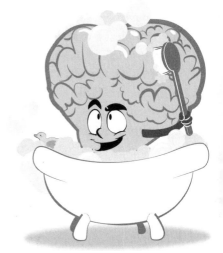

I'm going to wash that lead right out of my head…

Conventional medicine does not typically connect brain disorders with toxicity, except in conditions that are overt and cause damage, such as acute lead or mercury exposure. However, mounting research is beginning to reveal that lower-level toxic exposures may accumulate over time to cause slow degeneration of brain and nervous system tissue.

Heavy Metal Toxicity

Toxic metals such as aluminum, arsenic, mercury, cadmium, and lead are often referred to as heavy metals. These heavy metals from our environment are capable of accumulating in the body, especially in the brain, liver, kidneys, bones, and immune system. Most of the heavy metals in the body are a result of contamination from industry.

Sources of heavy metal toxicity include:

- **Aluminum** – aluminum-containing antacids, aluminum foil or cookware, drinking water
- **Arsenic** – drinking water, rice products
- **Cadmium** – cigarette smoke, drinking water
- **Lead** – car exhaust, dolomite, cosmetics, solder on tin cans, drinking water
- **Mercury** – dental amalgams (mercury fillings), drinking water, fish, shellfish

Signs and symptoms of heavy metal toxicity are usually vague. Mild cases may be associated with fatigue, headache, and "brain fog" (loss of concentration and clarity). More severe cases may involve chronic pain, tremors, anemia, dizziness, poor coordination, and other neurological symptoms.

According to a paper published by the National Institutes of Health, Americans have collectively lost 41 million IQ points as a result of exposure to lead mercury and organophosphate pesticides. Dr. David Bellinger, a professor of neurology at Harvard Medical School, calculates a total loss of 16.9 million IQ points in children due to exposure to organophosphates alone, the most common class of pesticides used in agriculture.

Heavy metals affect all three brains. Mercury, cadmium, and other heavy metals cause decreased oxidant defence and increased oxidative stress, affecting the heart brain and potentially leading to cardiovascular disease. Heavy metals and other toxins also cause leaky gut, leading to many health problems involving the three brains. (Refer to Chapter 2 for more information on leaky gut).

Environmental Toxins

Researchers report that environmental toxins are not just lowering IQ points, but they are also contributing to the increasing rates of autism spectrum disorder, attention deficit hyperactivity disorder (ADHD), and behavioural development disorders. The human brain, especially the developing brain, is especially susceptible to a variety of toxic chemicals. Various factors influence the brain's susceptibility to environmental toxins:

- The high fat content (60%) of the brain makes it particularly susceptible to long-term storage of fat-soluble toxic chemicals and free radical damage mediated by toxic chemicals, leading to increased tissue damage.

- Pesticides target delicate nerve tissue and promote free radical production, leading to inflammation.

- Sulphur-containing amino acids in the brain react readily with common toxic metals like mercury, cadmium, and lead, making the brain a vulnerable target for these chemicals. The sulphur amino acids not used for protein synthesis are used for the production of glutathione, which serves as a potent antioxidant for thousands of environmental chemicals. Exposure of the brain to these chemicals results in the depletion of glutathione, therefore diminishing the amount available for antioxidant duty and brain protection.

- Heavy metals and other toxic chemicals can cause inflammation in the three brains, making cells more vulnerable to a number of toxins.

Not being diagnosed with a learning disorder or a more severe degenerative neurological condition does not mean that pesticides and other environmental toxins are not causing inflammation and oxidative damage in the brain that can eventually lead to bigger problems. Add this to the finding that other forms of stress and various stressors also cause inflammation, and it starts to look as if depression and other neurological disorders could be a kind of allergy to modern life – which might explain its ever-increasing prevalence around the world as we increasingly eat and stress ourselves into a state of chronic inflammation.

Defence against environmental toxins

N-acetyl-L-cysteine (NAC) is a precursor of both the amino acid L-cysteine and L-glutathione. As mentioned previously, exposure to environmental toxins results in the depletion of glutathione, thereby diminishing the amount available for antioxidant duty and brain protection. Historically, NAC has been used for chronic respiratory illnesses as well as an antidote for liver toxicity due to acetaminophen overdose. However, it is now emerging as a treatment for vascular and nonvascular neurological disorders.

More recently, animal and human studies of NAC have shown it to be a powerful antioxidant and a potential therapeutic agent in the treatment of heavy metal toxicity. NAC stimulates glutathione synthesis, promotes liver detoxification, and is a powerful free radical scavenger, therefore supporting the body during times of stress, infections, toxic assault, and inflammation.

Genetically Modified Organisms

According to an article by the David Suzuki Foundation, the first genetically modified crop was approved by the US Food and Drug Administration (FDA) in 1994. Since then, genetically modified corn, soy, sugar beets, and canola have become common local crops in Canada. In addition, genetically modified varieties of cottonseed oil, papaya, squash, and milk products are imported from the US into Canada. These crops – called Roundup Ready crops – have had their DNA altered to allow them to withstand the herbicide glyphosate (the active ingredient of Monsanto's herbicide Roundup). They are also known as glyphosate-tolerant crops. In only 20 years, genetically modified organisms (GMOs) have made their way into most of the processed foods available in Canadian grocery stores. Genetically modified apples, potatoes, and wheat are currently in the lineup for approval.

The safety of genetically modified foods is unproven, and a growing body of research connects these foods with several negative health effects, primarily the production of new allergens, antibiotic resistance, increased toxicity, decreased nutrition, and gluten-related disorders, including celiac disease, an autoimmune disorder. Canadian research published in the *Journal of Reproductive Toxicology* in 2011 identified the presence of pesticides associated with genetically modified foods in maternal, fetal, and non-pregnant women's blood.

Glyphosate enhances the damaging effects of food-borne chemical residues and environmental toxins. The negative impact on the body manifests as inflammation that damages cellular systems throughout the body and the brain. Several recent studies show that glyphosates are endocrine disruptors (chemicals that can interfere with the hormone system in mammals) that can cause developmental disorders, birth defects, and cancer tumours. Studies also link glyphosate to autism, Parkinson's, and Alzheimer's.

For these reasons, some developed nations have, at the very least, implemented policies requiring mandatory labelling of genetically modified foods, and some have issued bans on genetically modified food production and imports. Canada has not. Canadians are often unaware that the foods they choose contain GMOs.

Tips to avoid glyphosate:

- Eat organic foods – most are GMO free.
- Demand labelling of GMOs on all foods.
- Avoid food containing genetically modified glyphosate-tolerant foods.
- Do not use glyphosate chemicals on your lawns or gardens.

*The following foods **always** contain MSG: autolyzed yeast, calcium caseinate, gelatin, hydrolyzed proteins, monopotassium glutamate, sodium caseinate, textured protein, yeast extract, and yeast nutrient.*

*The following foods **often** contain MSG: flavouring, seasonings, soy sauce, soy protein, bouillon, malt extract, barley malt, anything enzyme modified, carrageenan, maltodextrin, pectin, protease, corn starch, citric acid, powdered milk, anything protein fortified, and anything ultra-pasteurized.*

Monosodium Glutamate and Food Additives

Monosodium glutamate (MSG) is a common food additive and flavour enhancer used commercially. Like many food additives, it has been linked to a variety of health problems, including obesity, food addiction, migraines, and other neurological conditions. Some researchers believe that MSG has toxic effects in the human body.

MSG is an excitotoxin, which means it overexcites brain cells to the point of damage or death, resulting in various degrees of brain damage and potentially triggering learning disabilities, migraines, autism, attention deficit disorders, seizures, hyperactivity, multiple sclerosis, Alzheimer's, Parkinson's disease, and Lou Gehrig's disease.

The good news is that people can make dietary changes and use natural supplementation to avoid MSG in order to help maintain optimal brain health and prevent many brain disorders.

Electromagnetic Fields

Many years ago, surgeon Robert Becker, MD, said that "Our bodies and brains generate electromagnetic fields. We live in the earth's natural magnetic field and from the beginning we have been dependent on this environment. However we have now created a vast global network of man-made electromagnetic fields, the greatest polluting element in the earth's environment".

Prior to 2003, studies correlating cancer risk and cell phone use produced conflicting results. These results were based on studies of people who had used cell phones for three years on average, not long enough to develop cancer or other more serious brain disorders. The Environmental Working Group report, entitled *EWG's Guide to Safe Cell Phone Use*, reported the following in 2013:

- Analysis of all published cell phone brain tumour studies found that for people who had used a cell phone for 10 or more years, the overall risk for developing a glioma (a malignant brain tumour) increased by 90% on the side of the head where the cell phone was used. Researchers found the highest risk of brain tumours among people who started using cell phones during adolescence.

- A study showed 80% elevated risk for emotional and hyperactivity problems among young children who use cell phones and whose mothers also used cell phones during pregnancy.

- The National Research Council reported that exposure to cell phone radiation may affect the immune, endocrine, and nervous systems, fetal development, and overall metabolism.

- Multiple studies reported that the brains of young children absorb more radiation than those of adults (potentially rendering them more vulnerable to brain tumours). Scientists showed that under standard conditions of use, twice as much cell phone radiation would penetrate a child's thinner, softer skull than an adult's, and children will be exposed to cell phone radiation for more years and therefore in greater total amounts than the current generation of adults.

- One of the larger studies by the International Agency for Research on Cancer explored whether or not cell phones and brain tumours, specifically meningioma and glioma, were linked. The results were inconclusive.

There were suggestions of an increased risk of glioma at the highest exposure levels, but biases and error prevented a causal interpretation.

In spite of the research, the scientific community remains at odds over the issue of whether cell phone use is linked to health issues, partly because it takes years for cancers to develop. However, Health Canada suggests that consumers should:

- Limit the length of cell phone calls.

- Replace cell phone calls with text messages or use "hands-free" devices.

- Encourage children under the age of 18 to limit their cell phone usage.

In addition, to limit exposure to radio waves and electromagnetic fields (EMFs) emitted by cell phones and base towers, AM-FM transmitters, and TV broadcast signals, follow these tips:

- Do not use a microwave.

- Don't wear your cell phone like a pager. If your phone is turned on and worn on your belt or in a pocket you could be receiving a constant blast of radiation from the battery pack. Carry your cell phone in your purse or briefcase to minimize exposure.

- Minimize your time in front of the TV and computer.

Germany, Switzerland, Israel, the United Kingdom, France, and Finland, along with the European Parliament, have recommended actions to help consumers reduce exposure to cell phone radiation, especially for young children. US federal agencies that regulate cell phones, the FDA, and the Federal Communication Commission (FCC), have all but ignored evidence that long-term cell phone use may be risky. The FCC adopted radiation standards developed by the cell phone industry 17 years ago. These standards, still in use, allow 20 times more radiation to reach the head than the rest of the body. They do not account for risks to children.

While Health Canada sets exposure limits for radio-frequency electromagnetic energy from wireless equipment in federal settings, it does not provide limits for the general public. The newest revisions to regulatory standards suggest slight restrictions to certain frequencies to ensure larger safety margins for all Canadians, including newborns and children.

Consumers need easy access to cell phone radiation information so that they can make informed purchasing decisions and protect themselves and their families from potential health concerns.

Prescription Medications

Many common prescription and over-the-counter medications can have negative effects on the brain by depleting the nutrients required to protect the brain from inflammation and free radical damage. The list of pharmaceuticals that have negative effects on the brain is extensive. Following are some of the nutrients that can be affected by commonly prescribed medications.

Coenzyme Q10

Coenzyme Q10 (CoQ10) is a fat-soluble antioxidant that protects the brain from free radical damage and inflammation. It is essential for the production of the fuel used by cells to produce energy, adenosine triphosphate. If you become depleted in CoQ10, your brain will be sluggish and tired, memory and learning ability will be diminished, and there is increased risk for brain disorders. If your brain is low on energy it cannot make the required neurotransmitters, the messengers that help your brain neurons communicate.

Please note that the FDA released new safety information for statins, stating that cognitive impairment, such as memory loss, forgetfulness, and confusion have been reported by some statin users.

Some of the commonly prescribed drugs that lower CoQ10 include: beta blockers used to lower blood pressure; antidiabetic drugs; anticholesterol drugs (statins); diuretics; and antidepressants, especially the tricyclics (doxepin, amitriptyline, and imipramine).

If you are taking medications that deplete CoQ10, take a daily supplement.

B vitamins

The B-complex vitamins are essential for optimal brain function. Deficiency of any one of the eight B vitamins can affect how you think, feel, and behave. The B vitamins are water-soluble and easily excreted, so they need to be replenished daily. Each B vitamin has different functions in the brain and nervous system. Vitamin B deficiency can result in elevated levels of the amino acid homocysteine. Research links poor performance on mental function tests to elevated homocysteine levels. Elevated homocysteine levels also increase the risk for depression, Alzheimer's, vascular dementia, heart disease, and stroke. B vitamins are critical for mood regulation and concentration, and a deficiency of B12 can cause severe confusion and brain fog at any age. Vegetarians are typically deficient in vitamin B12.

Common medications that deplete B vitamins include, but are not limited to, oral contraceptives, estrogen, aspirin, antacids, antidiabetic drugs, blood pressure lowering drugs, asthma drugs, statins, nonsteroidal anti-inflammatory drugs (NSAIDs), and corticosteroids. In addition, antibiotics deplete all B vitamins, as well as bifidobacteria and lactobacillus, the good microbiota in the gut. If you are taking any of these medications, add a high-potency B-complex vitamin or a high-potency multivitamin to your daily vitamin regime.

Vitamin D

Vitamin D is associated with a significant increased risk for dementia and Alzheimer's. It can be depleted by antacids, antidepressants, statins, and gout medications (colchicines).

Glutathione

Glutathione, a very important protective antioxidant in the brain, was mentioned earlier. Aspirin, acetaminophen, ibuprofen, naproxen, and environmental toxins deplete levels of glutathione. If you take any of these medications on a regular basis, consider adding N-acetyl-L-cysteine (NAC) to protect the brain from glutathione depletion.

Tests to Help Save Your Head and Heart Brains

While there may not be a definitive test for most brain disorders, a range of tests can help identify possible risk factors, allowing for early intervention and treatment. Tests for inflammation and cardiovascular disease should be considered as risk factors for cognitive decline. Tests that can help save your head and heart brains include:

- **C-reactive protein (CRP)** – The most common test used to detect levels of inflammation in the bloodstream measures a substance called CRP. The body makes CRP from the pro-inflammatory cytokine interleukin-6 (IL-6), produced mostly by the liver. Over the past decade, an improved test, the highly sensitive CRP (hs-CRP) test, became available. CRP is a risk factor for cognitive impairment and dementia.

- **Oxidata** – This test is usually performed by a naturopathic doctor. It assesses free radical burden in the body, which can lead to chronic inflammation.

- **Lp-PLA2 (PLAC)** – This test measures Lp-PLA2, an enzyme that promotes inflammation inside the arteries, leading to the formation of unstable, rupture-prone plaques. Phospholipase A2 (PLA2) is a key enzyme in the metabolism of membrane phospholipids that also influences the processing and secretion of the amyloid precursor protein, which give rise to the beta-amyloid peptide, the major component of the amyloid plaque in Alzheimer's.

- **Homocysteine** – This common amino acid is related to early development of heart and blood vessel disease. A high level of homocysteine causes inflammation in the blood vessels, which in turn may lead to atherosclerosis, thereby increasing the risk factors for blood clots, heart attacks, and strokes, as well as cognitive problems.

- **Heavy metal testing** – Heavy metal toxicity of lead, mercury, aluminum, and cadmium can increase inflammation and cause damage to delicate brain tissue.

- **Fasting blood sugar and insulin** – Diabetes, metabolic syndrome, and insulin resistance can all increase the risk of cognitive decline and some brain disorders.

- **Blood pressure monitoring** – Hypertension has been linked to cognitive decline and memory problems, even in young adults.

- **Thyroid hormones** – These tests are used to determine either hyperthyroid or hypothyroid conditions. Typically only TSH (thyroid stimulating hormone) is tested, however it is important to also test for the thyroid hormones free T3, free T4, reverse T3, as well as thyroid antimicrosomal antibodies (TPO Abs) and antithyroglobulin antibodies (Tg Abs).

- **Salivary cortisol** – This test is used to determine clinical or preclinical adrenal dysregulation. It can be done through a naturopathic doctor or an alternative medical doctor.

- **Hemoglobin A1C** – This protein in the red blood cell carries oxygen and binds to blood sugar. It is typically tested to help determine the risk for diabetes, as it increases as blood sugars become elevated. Elevated A1C has been linked to Alzheimer's and mild cognitive impairment, increased risk of depression, and changes in brain size.

- **Allergy tests** – Enzyme-linked immunosorbent assay (ELISA) is used to test both IgE and IgG allergy reactions.

- **Apolipoprotein E (ApoE4)** – This protein is measured to test for genetic risk for Alzheimer's disease, particularly in women.

- **Single-photon emission computerized tomography (SPECT) scan** – This test indicates the amount of blood flow in the capillaries of the imaged regions. Some health care practitioners are using SPECT scans to help diagnose mental health disorders. The general consensus is that SPECT scans are valuable for a number of neurologic disorders, such as seizures, head injuries, dementia, and brain tumours. This method of diagnosis for various brain disorders such as depression, addiction, learning disorders, etc. is not commonly accepted by health care practitioners in the field of neuropsychiatry. However, when new concepts and methods are introduced, it takes time – often many years – for them to be accepted into mainstream thinking. For example, Dr. Daniel Amen, a psychiatrist in the US and medical director of Amen Clinics, uses SPECT scans to assess different brain disorders and focuses on nutritional supplementation to balance these various disorders when possible, as opposed to pharmaceutical treatment. His approach is helping thousands of people who previously had no success with conventional talk therapy or pharmaceutical intervention.

- **Positron emission tomography (PET) scan** – This test can help detect functional abnormalities early in the course of the disease, before anatomical changes occur. Brain disorders start with functional abnormalities that result in either an increase or decrease in glucose metabolism at a cellular level. These functional changes precede the formation of an abnormal mass, the shrinkage of brain tissue, or other abnormalities, sometimes by years.

A multitude of factors, including the brain busters mentioned in this section, can influence brain function. Individuals can also do many things to prevent and/or treat damage to this delicate three-brain orchestra. Section 3 provides information on how diet, lifestyle, and natural health supplements can help promote optimal health on all levels.

Creating Optimal Health

"The doctor of the future will give no medicine, but will interest his patients in the care of the human frame, in diet, and in the cause and prevention of disease." – Thomas Edison

What Is Optimal Health?

What are the basic steps required to create overall optimal health? The first step is knowing what optimal health is. Optimal health is more than the absence of disease or the suppression of symptoms. When we are experiencing optimal health, we enjoy a vibrant sense of well-being on all levels: physical, emotional, mental, and spiritual. We are in a state that promotes optimal function, regeneration, and repair of the body's cells, tissues, and organ systems. Once we understand what we are trying to achieve, then we will be in a position to more readily assess the ability of different medical approaches, based as they are on distinct philosophies, to meet our needs. We will also be able to make more informed choices regarding health promotion and disease prevention, as well as treatment options.

When patients are asked why they are taking a certain prescription medication, most do not know. They are simply following their doctor's orders. However, doing what you are told to do without understanding why you are doing it often does little to change a situation. Instead, ask questions, know your options, and make sure you are comfortable with your decision. Medical doctors, in many cases, are not used to having their authority questioned and may become annoyed at your questioning. Yet the word "medical doctor" does not mean "medical deity". It comes from the Latin docere, which means to teach.

When you blindly follow the directions of others, based only on their attitudes or opinions, your life can become a puppet show of sorts. The alternative is to become the "cause" of events in your life – to make informed choices. Once you choose to become the cause in your life, and more specifically in your health care, you will see that you always have options and choices.

The Master Tuners of the Three-Brain Orchestra

Tuning the main players in the three-brain orchestra is the secret to achieving an optimal performance. Fuel for the three brains starts with a good diet and lifestyle, and added supplements provide the necessary building blocks for the brain. For example, carbohydrates are required for energy; proteins for the synthesis of neurotransmitters; antioxidants to prevent free radical damage and inflammation; and good fats to build and protect healthy brain cells. Finally, water is the often-forgotten nutrient that is critical for tuning of the three brains.

Accumulating evidence suggests that diet and lifestyle play a vital role in maintaining and improving brain function, delaying the onset or halting the progression of many brain disorders, and improving cognitive function in general. This is not an alternative approach, it is fundamental: nutrition matters.

Energy and the Brain

The human brain is highly metabolically active and it depends on a constant supply of glucose to meet its energy needs. In fact, the brain uses at least 25% of total body glucose despite representing only 2% of adult body weight. The main fuel for all the body's cells, including the brain's, is glucose. However, eating more sugar for fuel is not the answer, as refined sugars end up causing rapid fluctuations in blood sugar, resulting in mental symptoms including depression, anxiety, irritability, dramatic mood swings, confusion or forgetfulness, and difficulty concentrating. Over time, blood sugar dysregulation commonly leads to metabolic syndrome and diabetes, factors in many brain disorders. Sugar consumption is a main contributor to the gut brain disorder called dysbiosis, which causes gastrointestinal disorders as well as many mental emotional symptoms. (Refer to Chapter 2 for more information on dysbiosis.)

The United States Department of Agriculture (USDA) reports that the average American consumes 68–77 kg (150–170 lb) of refined sugars in one year. That is equivalent to consuming 125–250 g (0.25–0.50 lb) of sugar each day, or 30–60 tsp of sugar in a 24-hour period. That is a lot of sugar, especially when you compare it to how much we used to consume. Less than 100 years ago, the average intake of sugar was only about 1.8 kg (4 lb) per person per year.

However, US consumption patterns do not accurately reflect Canadian sugar intake. Added sugar consumption in Canada is about one-third less than in the

US, due in part to our lower soft drink consumption. It only takes four 355 mL (12 oz) cans of soft drink to equal 125 g (0.25 lb) of sugar. US consumption of soft drinks is double that of Canada. However, even though our rates are lower, the average sugar intake in Canada is still 22–26 kg year (50–56 lb), which is too much sugar.

How to Control Blood Sugar Swings

The glycemic index (GI) measures how quickly blood sugar increases after eating a particular food: the higher the GI, the faster the rise and more rapid lowering of blood sugar. Foods with a high GI, such as refined sugars, white flour products, and other sources of simple carbohydrates and sugars, are quickly absorbed into the bloodstream. As a result, it is important to avoid junk food and pay more attention to the GI of the food you eat by choosing foods in the low to medium GI categories. Table 5.1 shows the GI of a variety of common foods.

Table 5.1 Glycemic Index of Foods

FRUIT AND VEGETABLES		
LOW	**MEDIUM**	**HIGH**
Green vegetables	Yams/sweet potatoes	Potatoes
Brassica family	Raw carrots	Beets
Tomatoes	Blueberries	Parsnips
Apples	Grapes	Dried fruit
Pears	Orange juice	Pineapples
Cherries		Bananas
Grapefruit		Raisins
Peaches		Mangoes
Beans (lentils, black, mung, pinto, black-eyed, chickpeas)		
GRAINS		
LOW	**MEDIUM**	**HIGH**
Pearl barley	Corn	Couscous
Rice bran	Brown rice	English muffin
Whole rye	Oat bran/oatmeal	French baguette
Wheat bran	Wild rice	Bread

Quinoa	Pumpernickel	Millet
Slow Oats		Crackers
		Taco shells
		Corn flakes
		Rice krispies
		Shredded wheat

PGX®

In addition to diet and exercise, PGX, a healthy fibre supplement that keeps the gut brain happy, can be very beneficial in preventing blood sugar swings and metabolic disorders that contribute to many different mental health conditions. PGX (PolyGlycopleX®) is a completely new and unique fibre matrix. The effectiveness of any fibre for reducing appetite, regulating blood sugar, and lowering cholesterol is based on the amount of water the fibre is able to absorb. The health benefits linked to soluble dietary fibre, including stabilizing blood sugar levels, are significantly magnified with PGX. For more information on the benefits of PGX please refer to www.pgx.com.

Detailed published clinical studies indicate that PGX has the following benefits:

- Stabilizes blood sugar in overweight and obese persons
- Reduces appetite and promotes weight loss, even in the morbidly obese
- Increases insulin sensitivity and decreases blood insulin levels
- Improves diabetes control
- Lowers blood cholesterol and triglycerides

Dosage: 750–1500 mg before each meal. Supports the three brains.

For weight loss: 2500–5000 mg before meals (start with a dosage of 750–1000 mg and work your way up to the full dosage over the course of two weeks).

Chromium Picolinate

Chromium picolinate also helps stabilize blood sugar. Those who experience symptoms of hypoglycemia should consider adding it to their supplement regime.

Dosage: 200 mg 1–2 times daily.

(Refer to Chapter 7 for more information on blood sugar dysregulation and mood swings.)

From Proteins to Neurotransmitters

Proteins provide the amino acids used to make neurotransmitters, including dopamine, serotonin, gamma-aminobutyric acid (GABA), and acetylcholine. Some of these amino acids are essential, meaning that the body does not make them and they must be provided by our diet. These amino acids are: lysine, tryptophan, methionine, valine, leucine, isoleucine, histidine, threonine, and phenylalanine. Figure 5.1 shows the amino acid precursors for specific neurotransmitters.

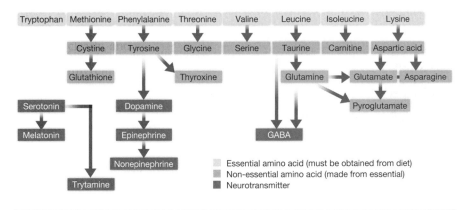

Figure 5.1 Amino Acid Precursors for Neurotransmitters

Neurotransmitter Building Blocks

Meat, fish, poultry, dairy products, and eggs are complete proteins containing all of the essential amino acids. Legumes, nuts, and seeds also provide sources of amino acids, but most are incomplete and need to be combined in order to provide the necessary amino acid building blocks to make protein. An example would be to combine rice with lentils.

Commercially produced meats are fed with grains like soy beans and corn, a diet that is high in inflammatory omega-6 fatty acids, but low in anti-inflammatory omega-3 fatty acids. Due to their small and tight living environment, these animals also gain excess fat and end up with high saturated fats. In contrast, organic free-range animals that are fed a natural diet such as grasses, instead of grains and hormones, have more omega-3 fatty acids. Having more room to roam freely, they are also leaner and contain less saturated fats. You may recall the role of inflammation as a cause of many brain disorders.

In addition to proteins obtained from the diet, a good quality protein powder added to blender drinks in the morning can be a good source of amino acids. Table 5.2 outlines the foods and supplements that support neurotransmitter health. (Refer to Chapter 1 for more information about individual neurotransmitters.)

Table 5.2 Food and Supplements to Support Neurotransmitters

DOPAMINE BUILDERS

Building blocks: tyrosine and phenylalanine

Foods: beef, chicken, turkey, eggs, oats, cottage cheese, and yogourt

Supplement support: B complex, B6, rhodiola, phosphatidylserine, methionine, and ginkgo biloba

SEROTONIN BUILDERS

Building block: tryptophan

Foods: avocado, chicken, chocolate, cottage cheese, eggs, milk, turkey, yogourt, and wholegrain carbohydrates

Supplement support: 5-HTP, fish oils, B1, B2, B6 vitamin D, folic acid, calcium, and magnesium tryptophan

GABA BUILDERS

Building block: glutamine

Foods: beans, corn, legumes, fish, meat, poultry, brown rice, wild rice, root vegetables, whole grains, almonds, walnuts, bananas, and green tea

Supplement support: GABA, B1, B3, B6, melatonin, and inositol

ACETYLCHOLINE BUILDERS

Building block: choline

Foods: almonds, beef, poultry, blueberries, broccoli, cabbage, eggs, pine nuts, hazelnuts, and cheeses

Supplement support: phosphatidylcholine, GPC choline, phosphatidylserine, huperzine-A, L-carnitine

Omega-3 Fatty Acids and the Three Brains

Ashes to ashes, dust to dust, oil those brains before they rust.

The human brain is nearly 60% fat, and essential fatty acids (EFAs) are among the most crucial nutrients that determine the brain's optimal function. Omega-3 fats are polyunsaturated fats. There are three main omega-3s: eicosapentaenoic acid (EPA), docosahexaenoic acid (DHA), and gamma-linolenic acid (ALA). They cannot be synthesized by the body and therefore must be obtained from dietary sources.

The omega-3 fatty acids are involved in the synthesis and function of brain neurotransmitters. They are highly concentrated in the brain and are important for general brain function. Brain disorders that have been linked to a deficiency of EFAs include dementias, depression, mood swings, brain fatigue, poor memory, and learning disorders.

Omega-3 Fatty Acids and the Head Brain

Research results on the role of EFAs and head brain health include the following:

- In a study published in September 2011 in the *British Journal of Nutrition,* the groups that received fish oil rich in the omega-3 components EPA and DHA for six months had improved scores on the Geriatric Depression Scale, but the results were more pronounced in the DHA group. "These results indicate that DHA-rich and EPA-rich fish oils may be effective for depressive symptoms and health parameters", the researchers wrote.

- Research published in August 2011 in the *Journal of Clinical Psychiatry* found a link between DHA and suicide. US scientists compared routine blood samples taken from 800 army service members who committed suicide between 2002 and 2008, and compared them to 800 other service members. The researchers found that men with the lowest levels of DHA were 62% more likely to commit suicide.

- In a study from the University of California, Los Angeles (UCLA), researchers found that rats fed a fructose-rich and omega-3 fat-deficient diet (similar to what is consumed by many Americans) developed both insulin resistance and impaired brain function in just six weeks.

- Several studies have shown that omega-3 fatty acids have a positive effect on neurons in the brain as well as antioxidant and anti-inflammatory activity. The mechanism of polyunsaturated fatty acids (PUFAs) in the brain provide a basis for mood regulation, cognitive function, and are beneficial in the treatment of depression, anxiety and social anxiety disorders, bipolar disorder, as well as ADHD.

Omega-3 Fatty Acids and the Heart Brain

The active constituents of fish oils, DHA and EPA, have anti-inflammatory effects. The EPA component has especially potent anti-inflammatory properties beneficial for inflammatory conditions of both the heart brain and the head brain. The DHA component is an important structural component of the head brain, eyes, and nervous system.

Canadian researchers examined the effects of daily ingestion of ground flaxseed on systolic (SBP) and diastolic blood pressure (DBP) in patients with peripheral artery disease. Individuals with a baseline SBP greater than 140 mm Hg who consumed 30 g of flaxseed daily for six months obtained an average reduction of 15 mm Hg in SBP and 7 mm Hg in DBP, while those with normal BP showed no effect. This study shows that the simple addition of flaxseed to the diet produces a potent blood pressure-lowering action in people with high BP.

Omega-3 Fatty Acids and the Gut Brain

Gut microbiota regulate gut motility, gut barrier homeostasis, and fat distribution. Since fatty acids play an important role in shaping gut microbiota metabolism, it is unsurprising that they have been considered as a dietary means to impede cognitive decline in aging. (Refer to Chapter 1 for more information on gut microbiota.) Human and animal studies on omega-3 fatty acids show heart and head brain protective roles through reducing inflammation and oxidative stress.

The typical North American diet tends to contain 14–25 times more omega-6 fatty acids than omega-3 fatty acids; omega-6 is pro-inflammatory, while omega-3 is anti-inflammatory. Omega-3 DHA and EPA are primarily found in fish oils such as herring, salmon, mackerel, sardines, and halibut, while ALA is primarily found in flaxseed oil, soybeans, walnuts, and green leafy vegetables, as well as in some animal fats, especially grass-fed animals. Omega-6 fatty acids (linoleic acid) are found in almond oil, peanut oil, Brazil nut oil, pecan oil, canola oil, pumpkin seed oil, evening primrose oil, safflower oil, flaxseed oil, sesame seed oil, grape seed oil, sunflower seed oil, walnut oil, and coconut oil.

Omega-3 Fatty Acid Recommendations

In addition to consuming foods rich in omega-3 fatty acids such as flaxseed, EFA supplements are highly recommended to help support optimal brain health. When choosing an EFA product, ensure it is free from heavy metals such as lead and mercury, as well as pesticides and other contaminants. Look for a combined product containing EPA and DHA from anchovy, sardine, or mackerel.

Dosage: 1000 mg combined EPA/DHA daily for general health; 3000 mg daily for inflammatory conditions.

Note: Omega-3 fatty acids should be used cautiously by people who bruise easily, have a bleeding disorder, or take blood-thinning medications including warfarin (Coumadin), clopidogrel (Plavix), or aspirin.

Phospholipids and the Three Brains

Phospholipids (water-insoluble substances, or "lipids", that contain phosphorous) contribute to the development, differentiation, function, protection, and repair of the nervous system. They help synthesize acetylcholine and form the insulating layer (myelin) that covers the nerves. As a result of these actions, phospholipids enhance mood and mental ability, and protect from age-related memory decline and dementias, including Alzheimer's disease. Two of the main phospholipids are phosphatidylserine (PS) and phosphatidylcholine (PC).

Phosphatidylserine

There is increasing evidence that supplementation with PS can improve memory, mood, learning, and concentration, as well as specific brain disorders including seasonal affective disorder (SAD), depression, attention deficit/hyperactivity disorder (ADD and ADHD), and Alzheimer's. PS has also been shown to help people cope with anxiety, and stress-related mental health problems.

As a cornerstone for brain conservation programs, including attention to diet, lifestyle, and mental and physical exercise, PS has the potential to add years to our lives and life to our years.

"I've tested close to a hundred compounds for their effect on human memory, and phosphatidylserine (PS) is the most impressive one I've found so far." – Dr. Thomas Crook, *Nutrition Action Health Letter,* May 1997

(Refer to Chapter 9 for more information on the benefits of PS for memory and brain health.)

Phosphatidylcholine

Choline was officially recognized as an essential nutrient by the Institute of Medicine (IOM) in 1998 due to its wide-ranging roles in human metabolism. It is needed for neurotransmitter synthesis (acetylcholine), phospholipid synthesis (PC), lipid transport, and homocysteine reduction. A deficiency of acetylcholine is thought to be the most common cause for memory decline. Choline intake for children, men, women, and pregnant women is far below the adequate intake established by the IOM.

Choline deficiency interferes with the heart-brain axis and causes elevated levels of homocysteine, which has been associated with greater risk for cardiovascular disease and cognitive decline. In addition, deficiency of either vitamin B12 or folic acid can result in elevated plasma homocysteine concentrations. Research shows that subjects whose diets were rich in choline had the lowest levels of several inflammatory markers, including C-reactive protein, homocysteine, interleukin-6, and tumour necrosis factor. Remember the influence of inflammation on many neurological disorders.

Among the most concentrated sources of dietary choline are liver, eggs, peanuts, and wheat germ. Egg yolks are the most concentrated source, providing 125 mg in one large egg. Meat, poultry, fish, dairy foods, rice, spinach, beets, and shellfish are also good sources of choline. PC, which contains about 13% choline by weight, is the main form of choline in dietary supplements. Pure choline has a very fishy smell and this can be off-putting for some, so PC may be preferred.

Phospholipids are required daily to maintain optimal brain function, so it is wise to add choline-based supplements in addition to food sources. Excellent sources of supplemental choline include PC, which is found in lecithin and which readily crosses the blood-brain barrier; alpha-glycerophosphorylcholine (Alpha-GPC), which is a potent form of choline derived from soy lecithin; and high-PC lecithin.

 LOOK for a product such as...

Brilliant Mind, which contains omega-3 fatty acids, phosphatidylcholine (PC), phosphatidylserine (PS), alpha-glycerophosphorylcholine (Alpha-GPC), and green tea extract.

Trans Fats and the Three Brains

In 2009, the World Health Organization (WHO) declared that trans fats were toxic, and sensible countries have since banned them. These artificial plastic fats increase the risks for inflammation, obesity, type 2 diabetes, insulin resistance, cardiovascular disease (CVD), and mental health disorders including depression, anxiety, memory problems, irritability, and aggression.

Trans fats are in any product that has partially hydrogenated vegetable oil, which is prominent in margarine and commercially-prepared baked goods and snacks. Trans fats compete with EFAs needed for the brain and general health.

Antioxidants for Three-Brain Defence

Antioxidants are chemicals that break down or neutralize the damaging effects of free radicals, which are chemicals produced as a by-product of normal cellular metabolism. Free radicals are destructive in that they cause oxidative damage to tissues. They damage proteins, fat, and even our DNA. The human brain is at particularly high risk for damage by free radicals because of its high degree of metabolism compared to other tissues, while lacking the levels of antioxidant protection found elsewhere in the body. Excessive free radical damage is now thought to be a major player not only in brain aging and traumatic brain injury, but in degenerative conditions like Alzheimer's as well as mild cognitive impairment. As cognitive function begins to decline, markers for free radical damage correlate directly with the degree of mental impairment.

An important key to enhancing antioxidant protection lies in our DNA. High levels of free radicals turn on specific proteins in the cell's nucleus called Nrf2, which essentially open the door for the production of important antioxidants. Some of nature's most powerful Nrf2 activators include broccoli, turmeric, green tea, coffee, chocolate, and resveratrol, a chemical found in red wine. It is noteworthy that epidemiological studies have shown significantly less risk for Alzheimer's in cultures regularly consuming Nrf2 activators like turmeric and red wine. Researchers have shown that an antioxidant can delay the onset of all the indicators of Alzheimer's, including cognitive decline.

Antioxidant Research Findings

- Cacao *(Theobroma cacao)* is rich in flavanols, a type of antioxidant shown to facilitate brain cell connections and survival, and protect brain cells from toxins or the negative effects of inflammation. Cacao has also been shown to help lower blood pressure, improve blood flow to the brain and heart, prevent blood clots, and improve insulin resistance. In a study published in 2015 in the *American Journal of Clinical Nutrition,* older adults with mild cognitive impairment who consumed cacao flavanols every day for eight weeks made significant improvements in cognitive test performance that measured attention, executive function, and memory. A new study has shown that the consumption of dark chocolate can also reduce the effects of the stress hormones adrenaline and cortisol, thereby reducing the effects of stress on the body. Stress hormones are associated with many different brain disorders.

- Resveratrol is a plant compound, similar to the flavonoids in cacao, which shows some promise. A small clinical study showed that resveratrol improves memory and brain function, along with better hippocampus function and improved glucose metabolism. These are all positive factors for a healthy aging brain. Antioxidants rich in flavonoids include grapeseed, pine bark extracts, and curcumin.

- Green tea *(Camellia sinensis)* is a powerful antioxidant and neuroprotector that can modulate blood flow in the brain. In a recent study, EGCG – a key component of green tea – was found to promote the regeneration of brain cells and contribute to improved short-term and long-term memory. Green tea is associated with reduced mortality due to all causes, as well as mortality due to heart disease. Research also shows green tea reduces cholesterol and triglyceride levels, lowers blood pressure, reduces oxidative stress, and chronic inflammation.

- R-alpha-lipoic (ALA) acid can cross the blood-brain barrier to protect against oxidative stress in the brain. Examination of current research reveals protective effects in cerebral ischemia-reperfusion, amino acid brain injury, mitochondrial dysfunction, diabetes and diabetic neuropathy, genetic metabolic disorders, and other causes of acute or chronic damage to brain or neural tissue. Glutathione is a very important brain antioxidant, but when taken, it is broken down in the stomach before reaching the bloodstream. ALA is able to raise intracellular glutathione levels. ALA also is important in cell metabolism and is required for converting glucose into adenosine triphosphate (ATP) to produce energy inside cells. Preliminary human studies indicate that ALA is effective in numerous neurodegenerative disorders.

- N-acetyl-L-cysteine (NAC) stimulates glutathione synthesis, promotes liver detoxification, and is a powerful antioxidant. Recent studies have shown that it is a potential therapeutic agent in the treatment of cancer, heart disease, heavy metal toxicity, and other diseases characterized by free radical damage. NAC is thought to be of benefit in heart disease by lowering homocysteine and lipoprotein(a) levels, and it is now emerging as treatment for vascular and non-vascular neurological disorders including Parkinson's disease, tardive dyskinesia, some forms of epilepsy, multiple sclerosis, amyotrophic lateral sclerosis, and Alzheimer's. NAC can help facilitate recovery after traumatic brain injury and cerebral ischemia (Insufficient blood flow). These diverse clinical applications are linked to its ability to support the antioxidant systems during stress, infections, toxic assault, and inflammatory conditions.

The Gut Brain: Are Gut Microbiota the New Antioxidants?

Recently, attention has been given to the potential antioxidant role of gut microbiota.

Gut microbiota, also known as microflora, may contribute to antioxidant status in different ways:

- A recently published study found that most strains of gut microflora, especially bifidobacterium and lactobacillus, significantly increase levels of glutathione and superoxide dismutase. This is an exciting finding as these are important antioxidants that protect cells against free-radical damage.

- Preliminary research suggests that microflora are able to prevent the oxidation of the omega-3 fatty acid, linolenic acid. All cells are surrounded by lipid membranes, so free-radical damage can lead to cell dysfunction or death.

- Healthy gut microflora bind to harmful heavy metals and toxins and remove them from the digestive tract. The reduction of heavy-metal toxicity would lessen the chances for free-radical generation. Researchers also note the ability of gut flora to liberate antioxidants from the food we eat. By doing so, this is yet another way in which healthy gut flora help contribute to antioxidant status.

- Healthy gut flora help prevent an overabundance of harmful pathogens in the gut, lowering the risk of leaky gut.

While research in this area is just beginning, it appears that gut flora provide significant antioxidant protection and lessen the risk of developing a number of oxidative-based conditions like cardiovascular disease, as well as other inflammatory conditions.

Antioxidants and the Heart Brain

Atherosclerosis is a complex process involving the formation and buildup of plaque in the arteries. These plaques provide a barrier to arterial blood flow and may precipitate future cardiovascular events. Considerable evidence supports the key role of free radicals in the development of atherosclerosis. Low-density lipoproteins (LDLs), which undergo multiple changes in oxidation, are thought to promote atherosclerosis. Oxidation of LDL lipids leads to the production compounds that influence the functional integrity of vascular cells and increase circulating inflammatory cells. Antioxidants operate by inhibiting oxidation and free radical formation, and repairing oxidant-induced injury.

Magnesium and the Three Brains

Magnesium is an important mineral for more than 300 biochemical reactions in the body. Deficiency has been blamed for various symptoms, including arrhythmias, hypertension, ADHD, anxiety, seizures, leg cramps, restless legs syndrome, kidney stones, myocardial infarction, headaches, premenstrual syndrome, fibromyalgia, osteoporosis, altitude sickness, diabetes, fatigue, weakness, and other health problems.

A recent study by Health Canada showed that more than 34% of Canadians have a magnesium intake below the estimated average requirement and are at risk for various health problems associated with low magnesium. In addition, in 2009, the WHO published a report that stated that 75% of North Americans consume less magnesium than needed. Some say that we have a nationwide magnesium deficiency.

Magnesium deficiency results in cellular damage. Magnesium deficits are caused by stress hormones, excessive dietary calcium, as well as dietary deficiencies of magnesium. Case histories show rapid recovery (less than seven days) from major depression using 600–1200 mg daily. Magnesium has been found to be effective for treating depression, anxiety, insomnia, short-term memory loss, irritability, agitation, and headaches. The possibility that magnesium deficiency is the major cause of depression and other related mental health problems, as well as IQ loss and addiction, is enormously important.

My mother had dementia, and for the last few years of her life she was in a care home. One of the first things I noticed was that the elderly were never offered water, and as a result never drank water. Instead, they were given coffee and soft drinks or fruit juice. I felt that if I could just provide them with enough water, perhaps 40–50% of their physical or mental problems would resolve. One book that I recommend to all of my patients is *Our Body's Many Cries For Water* by F. Batmanghelidj, MD.

The Importance of Water

"Please drink – I need water to help me think!"

The brain is approximately 73% water and it depends on proper hydration to function optimally. Dehydration can impair short-term memory function and the recall of long-term memory. Negative effects of dehydration on cognitive performance have been shown in some, but not all, studies.

In our society we tend to focus on the findings from scientific studies. It is important to know that results can vary widely depending on the statistical analysis done by the various stakeholders and what outcome is desired. Sometimes, especially when it comes to something as basic as water consumption and brain health, it is better to just use common sense. A dehydrated, small, shrivelled up brain does not function as well as one that is well hydrated. Drink a minimum of 1.5–2 L (about 6–8 cups) of purified water daily.

Water balance in our bodies changes over time. The percentage of water compared to body mass may be as high as 75% in a newborn baby, but it progressively decreases over time to approximately 55% in elderly people. The thirst signals also become less sensitive as a person ages, and the elderly often do not recognize the need to drink water. In order to reduce the risks of mental decline with aging, it is wise to drink regularly, even when not thirsty, beginning in early middle age.

Eating for Optimal Health

The Mediterranean Diet

The Mediterranean diet is an excellent dietary guideline to follow. It emphasizes foods rich in omega-3 fatty acids, including whole grains, fresh fruit and vegetables, fish, olive oil, garlic, as well as moderate wine consumption. The traditional Mediterranean diet has shown tremendous benefit in fighting and preventing inflammation, heart disease, and cancer, as well as diabetes. It has the following characteristics:

- Olive oil is the principal source of fat.
- It centres on an abundance of plant-based foods, including fruit, vegetables, breads, pasta, potatoes, beans, nuts, and seeds.
- Foods are minimally processed and there is a focus on seasonally fresh and locally grown food.
- Fresh fruit is the typical daily dessert, with sweets containing concentrated sugars or honey consumed a few times per week at the most.
- Dairy products, principally cheese and yogourt, are consumed daily in low-to-moderate amounts and in low-fat varieties.
- Fish is consumed on a regular basis.
- Poultry and eggs are consumed in moderate amounts, about 1–4 times weekly, or not at all.
- Red meat is consumed in small, infrequent amounts.
- Wine is consumed in low-to-moderate amounts, normally with meals.

Good fats don't make you fat

A new study published in *Lancet* in June 2016 indicates that following a Mediterranean diet that is not calorie restricted and is high in healthy fats from olive oil or nuts does not cause weight gain compared with a low-fat diet. Fear of weight gain from highfat foods no longer needs be an obstacle to following a high-fat diet such as the Mediterranean diet, which is known to provide health benefits.

In addition to following a diet plan that holds closely to the Mediterranean diet, specific foods and supplements can help give your brain that extra boost.

Twelve Power Booster Foods for the Three Brains

1. Celery contains a compound called 3-n-butylphthalide (3nB) that has been shown to significantly improve learning deficits, as well as

long-term spatial memory. Researchers have concluded that 3nB shows promising preclinical potential as a multi-target drug for the prevention and/or treatment of Alzheimer's.

2. Eggs and meat are good sources of choline, a B vitamin known for its role in brain development and in improving cognitive function, learning, and memory.

3. Blueberries contain antioxidants and other phytochemicals that have been linked to improvements in learning, thinking, and memory, along with reductions in neurodegenerative oxidative stress. They are also relatively low in fructose compared to other fruit, making them one of the healthier fruit available.

4. Deep-water fish, such as wild salmon and other oily fish, are rich in omega-3 EFAs, which are essential for brain function. Omega-3s also contain anti-inflammatory substances. Consider eating one 115 g (about 4 oz) serving, 2–3 times a week.

5. Raw nuts and seeds are good sources of vitamin E. Higher levels of vitamin E correspond with less cognitive decline as a person ages. Add an ounce a day of walnuts, hazelnuts, Brazil nuts, filberts, almonds, cashews, peanuts, sunflower seeds, sesame seeds, flaxseeds, and unhydrogenated nut butters, preferably raw, such as peanut butter, almond butter, and tahini to your diet. A handful of pumpkin seeds every day provides the recommended daily amount of zinc, which is vital for enhancing memory and thinking.

6. Avocados are almost as good as blueberries in promoting brain health. Avocado is a fatty fruit, but it is a monounsaturated fat, which contributes to healthy blood flow, resulting in a healthier brain. Avocados also lower blood pressure. Because hypertension is a risk factor for decline in cognitive abilities, a lower blood pressure should promote brain health. Most researchers agree that the high levels of monounsaturated fat in avocado, especially oleic acid, play a role in these heart-related benefits. Nearly 68% of the fat found in one cup of avocado comes from monounsaturated, and olives contain similar levels. Avocados contain

phytosterols including beta-sitosterol, campesterol, and stigmasterol, which have anti-inflammatory benefits.

7. Beans stabilize glucose (blood sugar) levels. The brain is dependent on glucose for fuel. Since it cannot store the glucose, it relies on a steady stream of energy, which beans can provide.

8. Pomegranate juice offers potent antioxidant benefits, which protect the brain from the damage of free radicals. "Probably no part of the body is more sensitive to the damage from free radicals as the brain", says neurologist David Perlmutter, MD. He adds that citrus fruit and colourful vegetables are also high on the list of "brainy" foods because of their antioxidant properties – "the more colourful the better".

9. Freshly brewed tea, 2–3 cups daily, hot or iced, contains a modest amount of caffeine which can boost brain power by enhancing memory, focus, and mood. Tea also has potent antioxidants, especially the class known as catechines, which promotes healthy blood flow.

10. Dark chocolate has powerful antioxidant properties. It contains several natural stimulants, including caffeine, which enhances focus and concentration. It also stimulates the production of endorphins, which helps improve mood. One serving of 14–28 g (0.5–1 oz) daily will provide all the benefits you need.

11. Eat beets for the brain. Drinking beet juice increases blood flow to the brain in older people, a finding that suggests that beets may fight the progression of dementia. Beet roots contain high concentrations of nitrates, which are converted into nitrites by bacteria in the mouth. Nitrites help open blood vessels in the body by increasing blood flow and oxygen. Previous studies have shown that nitrites, also found in high concentrations in celery, cabbage, and other leafy, green vegetables like spinach, widen blood vessels. However, researchers say this was the first to find that nitrites also increase blood flow to the brain.

12. Red wine contains important antioxidants, called polyphenols, which are specifically beneficial in reducing the action of free radicals. Another substance found in red wine, although in fairly small amounts, is resveratrol, an antioxidant that tends to reduce LDL cholesterol and also may act to reduce inflammation and blood clotting. Even the alcohol content of red wine has some beneficial effects as well. It raises HDL, reduces LDL, and helps modulate blood pressure, when consumed in moderation. Spanish researchers recently

published a report in the *American Journal of Clinical Nutrition* in which they discovered that chronic consumption of red wine actually increases bifidobacterium in the gut of humans that is associated with reduction of inflammation and, as discussed earlier, is important in brain health.

Key Supplements for Three-Brain Health

Good nutritional status is the foundation for optimal function of the three brains and the maintenance of cognitive function at any age:

- In addition to various amino acids, the B vitamins are needed as cofactors for the synthesis of neurotransmitters for each brain. For example, B6 is a required coenzyme for the synthesis of several neurotransmitters including GABA, dopamine, norepinephrine, and serotonin.
- Vitamin C is required for synthesis of norepinephrine.
- Choline is a precursor for the neurotransmitter acetylcholine.
- Phenylalanine is a precursor for tyrosine, which then converts into dopamine, adrenaline, and noradrenaline.
- The minerals zinc, manganese, magnesium, and chromium are vital for brain health.

A good multivitamin and mineral supplement should include the necessary cofactors as well as antioxidants to support health and function of the three brains. In addition to vitamins and minerals, many supplements play a role in maintaining basic brain nutrition. While many nutrients are discussed throughout this book, the following supplements can be considered the foundation for supporting memory and concentration, and preventing cognitive decline.

Bacopa

Bacopa has been used for centuries to enhance memory and intellectual function, promote sleep, treat mild to moderate anxiety and depression, and promote longevity. It has been proven to facilitate adaptation responses and to normalize plasma cortisol in acute and chronic stress models. Stress is a major cause of inflammation and cognitive disorders. Bacopa is also an antioxidant and it has been proven to be neuroprotective and to improve cognitive performance, as well as reduce amyloid deposits in the brain. It also inhibits degenerative changes in the hippocampus, one of the brain's main memory-processing areas. Five randomized, double-blind, placebo-controlled trials provide evidence for its efficacy in improving cognitive performance in humans including: delayed-recall memory task, improved task reaction times, improved speed of information processing, learning rate, and memory consolidation, improved mental control, and retention of new information.

Dosage: 250–350 mg daily of a 30:1 extract standardized to 50% bacosides.

Ashwagandha

Ashwagandha has remarkable stress-relieving properties in addition to its excellent protective effects on the nervous system. Ashwagandha may be a promising alternative treatment for a variety of mental health problems such as anxiety and depression, as well as of degenerative neurological diseases such as Alzheimer's and Parkinson's disease. Stress, environmental toxins, and poor nutrition all have a detrimental impact on our nervous systems. Studies support ashwagandha's ability not only to relieve stress, but also to protect brain cells against cellular degeneration. In one of the most complete human clinical trials to date, researchers studied the effects of a standardized extract of ashwagandha on the negative effects of stress, including elevated levels of the stress hormone cortisol that causes many of the adverse effects of stress. The participants showed up to a 26% reduction of cortisol levels, a decline in fasting blood sugar levels, and improved lipid profiles. The participants reported increased energy, reduced fatigue, better sleep, and an enhanced sense of well-being.

Dosage: 125 mg once or twice daily of an 8:1 extract standardized to 8% withanolides.

Gingko biloba

Gingko increases blood flow to the brain and enhances memory. The antioxidant properties of gingko have been found to inhibit beta-amyloid plaques in Alzheimer's. Gingko has also been shown to lower risk of atherosclerosis and heart attack. It supports the head and heart brains.

Dosage: 150–250 mg daily of a 50:1 standardized extract.

Note: Contraindicated in people taking blood thinners such as Coumadin.

Phosphatidylserine (PS)

PS is an important phospholipid that can enhance mood and memory ability and protect from age-related memory decline and dementias, as well as Alzheimer's. (Refer to Chapter 9 for more information.)

Dosage: 100–300 mg daily.

Pyrroloquinoline quinone

Pyrroloquinoline quinone (PQQ) provides a wide range of benefits for healthy brain function, including antioxidant support and protection against the damaging effects of neurotoxins. Overall, PQQ helps prevent memory problems and cognitive decline.

Dosage: 20 mg daily.

Curcumin

Curcumin has potent anti-inflammatory and antioxidant properties that can help prevent and support inflammatory conditions. Research has shown that curcumin is comparable to common prescription medications like hydrocortisone and over-the-counter medications such as ibuprofen in the treatment of inflammation. Curcumin plays a significant role in the treatment of dementias, including Alzheimer's, as well as other brain disorders such as depression, and symptoms related to traumatic brain injuries. Research has demonstrated the ability of curcumin to cross the blood-brain barrier and bind and destroy the beta-amyloid plaques present in Alzheimer's. Curcumin also reverses chronic stress-induced behavioural, memory, and learning problems.

Dosage: 300 mg daily of a brand that has been optimized for maximum absorption.

Chamomile *(Chamomilla recutita)*

Chamomile has traditionally been used as a calming and anti-inflammatory herb and is sometimes called "herbal aspirin". More recent studies have shown that chamomile is effective in the treatment of depression and anxiety.

Dosage: 150 mg 3–5 times daily of a 4:1 extract.

Boswellia *(Boswellia serrata)*

Boswellia contains boswellic acids and has been used as a major anti-inflammatory agent for centuries. Many studies have shown that boswellia is just as effective as nonsteroidal anti-inflammatory drugs (NSAIDs), which are the most commonly used treatment for inflammation. Boswellia reduces post-injury inflammation and improves behavioural and cognitive dysfunction that result from traumatic brain injury and stroke, which are both common causes of dementia. Boswellic acids have also been found to stimulate the growth of neurons in the brain that support cognition and memory. Clinical trials show promising results supporting the anti-inflammatory effects of boswellia extract in patients with rheumatoid arthritis and osteoarthritis pain, chronic colitis, ulcerative colitis, Crohn's disease, atherosclerosis, bronchial asthma, and swelling in the brain. Preliminary animal studies also show that boswellia improves memory and learning abilities. The combination of boswellia and curcumin has proven more effective in the treatment of pain than most of the prescription drugs available for inflammatory disorders. In a four-month randomized study, one group received 100 mg of celecoxib twice daily, and the second group received a 500-mg blend of a curcumin extract and a boswellia extract twice daily. The efficacy and tolerability of the herbal combination was superior to that of the drug group in relieving pain, walking distance, and joint line tenderness scores.

Dosage: 400–800 mg daily of a standardized extract.

Fish oil

Omega-3 fatty acids are found in cold water fish and are involved in the synthesis of brain neurotransmitters. They are highly concentrated in the brain, and deficiencies have been linked to memory and cognitive problems as well as dementias. (Refer to Chapter 5 for more information on the importance of fish oils for brain health.)

Dosage: 1000–3000 mg daily.

CoQ10

Hypertension damages brain structures and leads to reduced cognitive ability and a greater risk for dementias. CoQ10 supports cardiovascular function and helps regulate blood pressure. (Refer to Chapter 5 for more information on how cardiovascular health affects cognitive ability and memory.)

Dosage: 50–150 mg daily.

Lutein

Although lutein is better known for its role in eye health, scientific evidence now indicates that lutein may be important for brain function as well. The brain is vulnerable to free radical damage due to its relatively low antioxidant levels and high concentration of fatty acids. Lutein functions as both an antioxidant and an anti-inflammatory agent and is therefore beneficial for those conditions where inflammation is a contributing cause, such as depression, memory problems, and cognitive disorders.

Dosage: 10–20 mg daily.

Grapeseed extract

Grapeseeds contains proanthocyanidin complexes, which are powerful antioxidants that destroy free radicals. Free radicals damage DNA and cause cell death, which contribute to aging as well as the development of a number of health problems, including heart disease and memory decline.

Dosage: 50–100 mg daily of an extract standardized to 80–85% oligomeric proanthocyanidins.

Prebiotics and Probiotics

Prebiotics are specialized plant fibres that nourish the good bacteria already in the large bowel or colon, while probiotics introduce good bacteria into the gut. Many studies confirm the benefits of fibre and probiotics for the prevention and treatment of mental health and neurological disorders, lowering cardiovascular risk factors, and many intestinal disorders. A strain such as BB536 contains *Bifidobacterium longum,* the most prevalent bacteria in the intestine.

Dosage: 1–2 capsules daily.

The Importance of Brain-Derived Neurotrophic Factor for Optimal Health

Neuroplasticity is the brain's ability to reorganize itself by forming new connections. This allows the nerve cells in the brain to compensate for injury and disease and to adapt in response to new situations and other changes in the brain. Neurotrophins support neuroplasticity by signalling nerve cells to differentiate or grow as well as influencing cellular metabolism. Exercise and training seem to be important in this process. Of all the neurotrophins, brain-derived neurotrophic factor (BDNF) is the most influenced by exercise.

BDNF has many functions in the brain and peripheral nervous system, including nerve cell protection and survival; growth and remodelling; and synaptic transmission. BDNF influences food appetite, increases oxidation of glucose, lowers blood glucose levels, and increases insulin sensitivity. In animals, it has been shown that a high-fat diet reduces the amount of BDNF in the hippocampus, but exercise is able to reverse this decrease.

Exercise and BDNF

In addition to the dietary components and nutritional factors necessary for a healthy brain, physical exercise as well as brain exercises are very important for optimal brain function. Exercise has been promoted as a possible prevention for neurodegenerative diseases. It has a positive influence on cognition and it increases BDNF, an essential neurotrophin. However, moderate exercise may be best. One study found that people who exercised as little as once and up to 30 times per month had higher levels of brain-protecting BDNF than non-exercisers or extreme exercisers. Exercise has also been shown to have positive anti-inflammatory benefits, which may promote both gut and brain health.

Nutritional Factors and BDNF

- Vitamin A is important for brain development. One study showed that mice deficient in zinc and vitamin A had low levels of nerve growth factor (NGF) and BDNF, while those on dietary supplementation had higher levels of both in the hippocampus, cortex, and cerebellum.

- Participants assigned to the Mediterranean diet plus nuts showed a significantly lower risk of low BDNF levels compared to the control group, and those with prevalent depression at baseline had significantly higher BDNF levels.

- Olive *(Olea europaea)* polyphenols are chemicals derived from plants known to possess antioxidant and anti-inflammatory properties. Various studies have suggested that dietary polyphenols may protect against cancer and cardiovascular, metabolic, and neurodegenerative diseases. One study in mice found that olive polyphenols may increase the levels of NGF and BDNF in crucial areas of the limbic system and olfactory bulbs, which play a key role in learning and memory.

- The influence of the gut microbiota on brain chemistry has been convincingly demonstrated in rodents. In the absence of gut bacteria, the expression of BDNF was reduced, whereas oral probiotics increase BDNF and also showed anti-anxiety effects. The researchers concluded that probiotics increase brain BDNF expression, possibly through the involvement of gut hormones. The data provide a sound basis for further investigation in the use of pre- and probiotics in the maintenance of brain health and adjunctive treatment of psychiatric disorders.

LOOK for...

Many excellent brain support supplements contain one or more of the above nutrients, but choosing which ones to take can be a challenge. For most people it is impractical to take a dozen or more individual supplements. On the other hand, combination formulas may not contain enough of any one ingredient to provide a benefit. One option is to look for a comprehensive "kit" that includes convenient daily packets. Each packet contains individual doses of the most essential supplements for basic brain health. Rather than purchasing each of the above-mentioned products individually, some brands offer a comprehensive "kit" that includes the most essential supplements for brain health in convenient daily packets. For example, **Daily Brain** includes phosphatidylserine-enriched sunflower (containing naturally occurring phosphatidylcholine [PC], phosphatidylinositol [PI], and phosphatidylethanolamine [PE]), curcumin, omega-3 fatty acids EPA and DHA, grapeseed extract, and key probiotic strains.

With the basics taken care of, additional supplements can be added based on individual needs. For example, since inflammation significantly contributes to many different disorders in all three brains, you may want to add an anti-inflammatory and cognition formula such as **Brain Defence,** which contains bacopa, ashwagandha, curcumin, boswellia, and chamomile.

The importance of phospholipids and omega-3 fatty acids to three-brain health was discussed earlier in this chapter, and you may want to take an additional dose of these key nutrients. Look for a product such as **Brilliant Mind,** that contains omega-3 fatty acids, phosphatidylcholine, phosphatidylserine, alpha-glycerophosphorylcholine, and green tea extract.

This chapter outlines some of the most important diet and lifestyle choices, along with key supplements, to support the health of the three brains. The following chapter outlines important nutritional factors for the developing brain.

Start Early to Protect the Developing Brain

Have you ever watched young children try to figure out the world around them? The developing brain is truly wondrous to behold. During the first three years of life, the brain is growing, growing, growing, and children absorb everything that is going on in their environment, as well as how to think, react, and talk, the meaning of words, and problem solving – like "How do I get that toy over there?" and "How do I stand up… crawl… walk… run?"

Activities like reading to your child, listening to music, building with blocks, doing puzzles, playing games, and exploring the surroundings encourage brain development. Nutrition is critical for healthy brain function in people of all ages, and even more in young children, adolescents, and teens as the brain is still growing and developing, as shown in Figure 6.1. For example by four years of age, a child's brain is more than twice as active as an adult's. The brain continues to consume glucose for energy and metabolism at high rates from 4–10 years of age, and then there is a gradual decline until age 16–18 when glucose use levels off at adult levels.

It is important to supply the developing brain with the building blocks it requires for high energy demands and growth, especially during these important periods of maximal learning capacity. Foods and supplements that contain antioxidants, essential fatty acids (EFAs), complex carbohydrates, and proteins are particularly helpful in boosting brain health. There is no guarantee that your children or teens are going to end up being another Einstein, but it is a smart start.

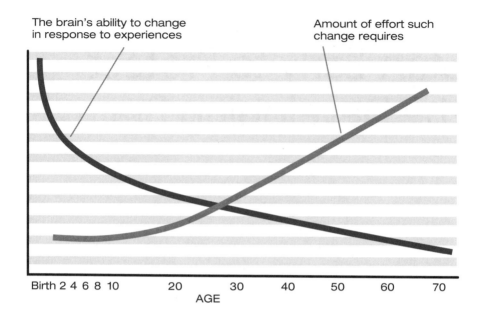

The brain's ability to change in response to experiences

Amount of effort such change requires

Figure 6.1 Brain development by age

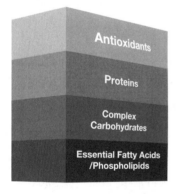

Fundamental Building Blocks of Brain Development

In general, the same ideas associated with healthy eating in adults apply to children. They require lots of fresh fruit and veggies, complex carbohydrates, complete proteins, good fats, and lots of water. If children turn their noses up at leafy greens, get a juicer and consider making vegetable juice with apples or carrots. It tastes good and should save time and lessen the arguments.

When it comes to fruit, focus on organic berries, a good source of polyphenols that are powerful antioxidants. In animal studies, researchers have found that blueberries in particular can help protect the brain, improve memory, promote neuroplasticity in the hippocampus, and improve insulin sensitivity.

Omega-3 Fatty Acids

Most children do not get enough omega-3 fatty acids in their diets. Studies clearly show that essential fatty acids (EFAs) are vital for optimal brain function in children. The omega-3 fatty acids are involved in the synthesis and functions of brain neurotransmitters. They are highly concentrated in the brain, and are important for brain memory and performance and behavioural function. Research findings demonstrate the importance of EFAs for brain development:

- Docosahexaenoic acid (DHA) is the most abundant omega-3 fatty acid in cell membranes in the brain. Studies have found that children who had below-average reading scores were particularly deficient in DHA and other omega-3 fatty acids. Moreover, children and teens with attention deficit hyperactivity disorder (ADHD) and related learning difficulties were more likely to have low EFA levels and could benefit from supplementation.

- Another study showed that DHA supplementation in early life increases intelligence as older children. In this case, infants received either an omega-3 fat supplement or a placebo. Cognition tests were given every six months starting at 18 months until the children were six years old. The group consuming omega-3 fatty acids consistently outscored the placebo group for 3–5 year olds. In general, the omega-3 group scored higher on rule learning, vocabulary, and intelligence testing. Because your brain is literally built from fatty acids, it makes sense that they play an integral role in brain function.

Only fish and krill contain both DHA and eicosapentaenoic acid (EPA) omega-3 fatty acids, which are crucial for brain function. Look for a supplement that has EPA and DHA derived from small fish (anchovy, sardine, and/or mackerel), providing at least 400 mg EPA and 250–300 mg DHA per capsule.

> I have three sons. When they were young, dinner was a battle of the wills as there would be endless arguments over eating vegetables. Eventually I came up with a plan and we arrived at an agreement. I made vegetable juice every dinner and the deal was that if they drank their juice before dinner, they didn't have to eat more vegetables with dinner. So basically they would plug their noses and down the juice… they got their vegetables and I got some peace.

Probiotics

The brain and microbes in the gut are vulnerable to damage during certain stages of development. The mother provides an infant's first bacterial exposure, thus maternal health is very important to how a child's microbiota environment develops. Maternal stress or infection during pregnancy has been linked to neurological and central nervous system disorders, such as schizophrenia, autism spectrum disorders, and distinct cognitive and behavioural symptoms later in life. The effects of the two-way relationship between stress and the gut microbiota may be at the root of this connection.

Antioxidants

Just to review: antioxidants are vitamins and other nutrients that help protect the cells from the damaging effects of free radicals. Free radicals are byproducts of digestion and toxins found in the environment that may contribute to many different health problems. (Refer to Chapter 4 for more information about free radicals.)

When teaching younger children about antioxidants, you may want to describe them as brain defenders or brain superheroes who fight the chemical bad guys that try to make you sick. The best sources of antioxidants are healthy, whole foods, such as brightly coloured fruit and vegetables. Bell peppers, berries, watermelon, red cabbage, sweet potatoes, and carrots are all examples of antioxidant-rich foods that children may enjoy seeing, touching, and tasting. Although the best way for younger children to get antioxidants is through diets high in fruit and vegetables, added supplementation can provide added insurance to protect the body and brain from oxidative stress and free radical damage.

A 2012 study conducted by the Centers for Disease Control and Prevention reported that at least 6% of North American children over the age of six may be deficient in vitamin C. According to the Food and Nutrition board, the intake level of vitamin C for adolescents should not exceed 1800 mg per day. For 9–13 year olds, 1200 mg is the acceptable limit, while 4–8 year olds should not exceed 650 mg. The first noticeable side effect of too much vitamin C is loose stool or diarrhea. Vitamin C is a water-soluble vitamin that is readily excreted by the body and does not cause harmful side effects. Humans do not make vitamin C in their body and must obtain it from food sources.

Unfortunately, most foods alleged to be high in vitamin C, such as citrus fruit, are sadly lacking due to early picking, shipping, and storage practices.

Multivitamins

A multivitamin and mineral for children helps provide necessary building blocks for a healthy brain that may be missing from the diet. A good quality multivitamin and mineral provides essential nutrients for the maintenance of good health. It provides vitamins A and C, both antioxidants, for added cell protection, and essential nutrients to help maintain eyesight, skin, and immune function, as well as promote the development of bones and teeth, and repair connective tissue.

Learning Disorders and ADHD in Children and Adolescents

ADHD is the most common disorder diagnosed in children. It affects 5–12% of school-aged children. Approximately 8–10% of males and 3–4% of females under age 18 have ADHD, and symptoms can continue into adulthood. The main behaviours associated with ADHD are inattention, hyperactivity, and impulsivity. Symptoms include difficulty staying focused and paying attention, difficulty controlling behaviour, and hyperactivity.

Most children get distracted, act impulsively, and struggle to concentrate at one time or another, and all children mature at different rates, have different personalities, and have different energy levels. Sometimes these normal factors may be mistaken for ADHD. ADHD symptoms usually appear early in life, often in children 3–6 years of age. Because symptoms vary from person to person, the disorder can be hard to diagnose and is becoming overly and wrongly diagnosed in many children. Anxious kids who are worried, preoccupied, and restless may also appear inattentive and unable to focus, but they don't necessarily have ADHD.

A University of British Columbia study published in the *Canadian Medical Association Journal* in March 2012 looked at the records of almost a million 6–12 year old children in the province of British Columbia from December 1997 to November 2008. The findings indicated a gradual increase in the treatment and diagnosis of ADHD. During the whole period, 6.9% of boys were diagnosed with ADHD and 5.5% were treated for it. For girls, the percentages were 2.2 and 1.6%, respectively.

Researchers were interested to see whether a relative age effect was present. They found that children were 39% more likely to be diagnosed and 48% more likely to be treated with medication for ADHD if born in December compared to January. Although generally the prevalence of ADHD diagnosis and treatment is about three times higher in boys than girls, when considering the age factor, girls born in December were 70% more likely to be diagnosed with ADHD than girls born in January. Due to the December 31 cut-off birth date for entry into school in British Columbia, children born in December would typically be almost a year younger than their classmates born in January.

The results show a relative age effect in the diagnosis and treatment of ADHD in children 6–12 years of age in British Columbia, raising concerns about the harms of overdiagnosis and overprescribing. These harms include sleep, appetite, and growth disruptions, in addition to increased risk of cardiovascular events and slower growth rates, as well as social stigma. Children who have been labelled as having ADHD may be treated differently by teachers and parents and peers, which could lead to negative self-perception and social and behavioural issues.

"The relative age of children is influencing whether they are diagnosed and treated for ADHD", said lead author Richard Morrow, University of British Columbia. "Our study suggests younger, less mature children are inappropriately being labelled and treated. It is important not to expose children to potential harms from unnecessary diagnosis and use of medications."

Diagnostic Criteria for ADHD

Although there is no definitive diagnosis for ADHD at this time, brain imaging studies have revealed that the brains of youths with ADHD mature in a normal pattern but are delayed, on average, by about three years. The delay is most pronounced in brain regions involved in thinking, paying attention, and planning. However, brain imaging is a new field in the diagnosis of mental health disorders and is not part of the standard diagnosis for ADHD or any other mental emotional disorder.

Many other factors affect learning ability. Younger children are often not able to articulate the feelings if there are other things going on in their life such as: a sudden change in the child's life such as the death of a parent; divorce; a parent's job loss; a move to a new city or school; undetected petit mal ("little illness") seizures where a child briefly loses and returns to consciousness; middle ear infections causing hearing loss; anxiety and depression; and more serious medical disorders that affect brain functioning.

Generally the diagnostic criteria for ADHD are based on a simple questionnaire. In some cases, a psychologist or other professionals in the field carry out an assessment, but this is usually not the case unless the case is more extreme.

In 2013, The American Psychiatric Association published DSM-V, the first major revision to the diagnostic manual for psychiatric disorders since 1994. To confirm a diagnosis of ADHD, individuals younger than age 17 must display at least six of nine inattentive and/or hyperactive impulsive symptoms. For individuals 17 years and above, however, only five or more symptoms are needed.

The nine inattentive symptoms are: (before each symptom include the word "often")

- Failing to give close attention to details or make careless mistakes in schoolwork, work, or during other activities
- Difficulty sustaining attention in tasks or play activities
- Unable to listen when spoken to directly
- Unable to follow through on instructions and failing to finish school work, chores, (e.g., starts tasks but quickly loses focus and is easily sidetracked)
- Difficulty organizing tasks and activities
- Reluctance to engage in tasks that require sustained mental effort
- Loses things necessary for tasks or activities
- Easily distracted by extraneous stimuli (for older adolescents and adults this may include unrelated thoughts)
- Forgetful in daily activities

The nine hyperactive/impulsive symptoms are:

- Fidgets with or taps hands or squirms in while seated
- Leaves seat in situations when remaining seated is expected
- Runs about or climbs in situations where it is inappropriate
- Unable to play or engage in leisure activities quietly
- "On the go" unable to be or uncomfortable being still for extended time
- Talks excessively
- Blurts out answers before questions have been completed
- Has difficulty waiting turn
- Interrupts or intrudes on others

Some children and adults have symptoms of both categories. Consider the symptoms listed above and ask yourself: What child or adolescent, or adult for that matter, does not exhibit five or six of these 18 symptoms?

The Importance of Movement

In a recent study, preteens and teens diagnosed with ADHD wore a device to measure activity levels. It was found that those who moved the most also showed the greatest accuracy in test results. The authors of the study published in the journal *Child Neuropsychology* suggested that the movement may be helping them focus and concentrate better. Another study done in younger children found the same results: those who moved the most performed best.

Movement is sensory-based and may help improve focus, increase alertness, and facilitate learning rather than interfering with the learning process. Previous research suggested that movement helps with cognitive function. When the brain is stimulated through physical movement, it reacts faster and with greater flexibility. This allows someone with ADHD to focus, retain information, and integrate concepts. Perhaps worming and squirming, leg-swinging, foot-bouncing, and pencil-tapping are actually important aspects of functioning for someone with ADHD. We don't know yet, but we know enough to be cautious about demanding that all children sit quietly and learn in the same way.

There are other forms of learning disorders and behavioural problems and there are overlaps between them. Dyslexia, dyspraxia, and ADHD all have varying degrees of severity and often overlap. People with dyslexia primarily have difficulty learning to read and write, while dyspraxia is difficulty with coordination. People with dyslexia are also likely to be dyspraxic and vice versa, and the cross-over between ADHD and dyslexia/dyspraxia is about 50%. Autism spectrum disorder is another brain disorder more commonly diagnosed in children today.

Some Causes of Learning Disorders and ADHD

External factors often significantly contribute to learning disorders. These include allergies or food intolerances, toxic exposure, stress, inflammation, blood sugar imbalances, thyroid disorders, overconsumption of sugar and re-fined carbohydrates, food additives like MSG, electromagnetic fields (EMFs), gluten intolerance, and dysbiosis and other gut microbiota imbalances. (Refer to Chapter 2 for more information.)

Gut and psychology syndrome

As discussed throughout this book, the gut microflora is a very important part of our human physiology. Recent research in Scandinavia has demonstrated that 90% of all cells and all genetic material in a human body consist of our own gut flora. Natasha Campbell-McBride, a doctor in the United Kingdom, developed the concept of the gut and psychology syndrome (GAPS). According to this model, the gut flora does not develop normally from birth in children with learning disorders such as autism, ADHD, ADD, dyslexia, or dyspraxia. As a result, the digestive system becomes a source of toxicity rather than a source of nourishment. The "bad" microbes damage the gut wall and toxins and microbes flow into the bloodstream, affecting the brain. Toxins prevent normal brain function and processing of information. In children who are breastfed, symptoms of different learning problems may occur around the second year of life because breast milk provides protection against abnormal microflora. In children not breastfed, problems may occur earlier.

Iron deficiency

In addition to the possible causes of learning disorders mentioned above, iron deficiency can cause a wide range of mood and behavioural abnormalities. In previous studies, a low serum ferritin (iron storage) concentration without anemia was found to be common in children with ADHD, with a prevalence as high as 84% in one study. Studies in general indicate that iron deficiency is an important contributing factor to ADHD in some children.

Children under two years of age and adolescents have higher iron requirements to support rapid growth. Their diet often proves inadequate and additional supplementation is required. Iron supplementation is suitable for children, although this should be done under the supervision of a health care practitioner to avoid excess iron levels and to monitor the effectiveness of supplementation.

Diet and EFAs

Considerable clinical and experimental evidence now supports the idea that deficiencies or imbalances in certain highly unsaturated fatty acids may contribute to a range of common developmental disorders, including ADHD, dyslexia, dyspraxia, and autistic spectrum disorders.

- A study from George Washington University found that ADHD symptoms in children receiving EFAs improved over children in control group receiving placebo. Another study found that hyperactive children who ate a meal high in protein did equally well or sometimes better in school than non-hyperactive kids.

- A recent special review article of more than 90 scientific publications summarized evidence of nutritional and dietary influences on ADHD, identifying suboptimal levels of certain nutrients in relation to behaviour and learning in children. Children with suboptimal levels of iron, zinc, and magnesium may demonstrate improvement in their hyperactivity and attention when supplemented appropriately with these nutrients.

- The results of additional studies indicated that supplementing ADHD children with omega-3 fatty acids was associated with improvement of their symptoms.

- The Oxford Durham study found that fatty acid supplementation may offer a safe and efficacious treatment option for educational and behavioural problems among children with developmental coordination disorder.

Food additives

In recent decades, our fast-paced life has led to changing lifestyles with increased demands for foods with a long shelf life that are easily prepared. Food additives, especially preservatives and artificial colours, as well as suboptimal intake of essential nutrients, have been linked to hyperactive behaviours and poor attention in many children. These risk factors have received little attention from the scientific community even though there is enough evidence to support these influences as risk factors. It is important to raise awareness among clinicians and, subsequently, review our food regulatory processes to better protect children in Canada.

"The biggest surprise of my research was the tremendously positive effect a simple change in nutrition had on children with ADHD", says Dr. Michael Lyon, a family physician and adjunct professor at the University of BC. Dr. Lyon's research repeatedly demonstrates the importance of the brain-immune-gut connection and how the food we eat not only nourishes the brain, but also poisons it. And, according to Dr. Lyon, most important are omega-3 fatty acids. Sensitive brains become dysfunctional when starved of them, especially if people have ADHD.

Parents and children are advised to limit unnecessary food additives and consume a diet rich in essential nutrients, and to be aware of the factors that contribute to learning disorders. For example, a double-blind placebo-controlled study of 137 three-year-old and 130 eight- or nine-year-old children from the general population supported the theory that artificial colouring and benzoate preservatives promote hyperactive behaviour in children. Experimental evidence indicated that common food additives, in combination, enhance neurotoxicity, providing support for their potential role in brain function and development.

Pesticides

A new study links a commonly used household pesticide with ADHD in children and young teens. The study found an association between pyrethroid pesticide exposure and ADHD, particularly in terms of hyperactivity and impulsivity, rather than inattentiveness. The association was stronger in boys than in girls.

Due to concerns about adverse health consequences, the United States Environmental Protection Agency banned the two most commonly used organophosphate (organic compounds containing phosphorus) pesticides from residential use in 2000–2001. The ban led to the increased use of pyrethroid pesticides, which are now the most commonly used pesticides for residential pest control. They are also increasingly used in agriculture.

"Given the growing use of pyrethroid pesticides and the perception that they may represent a safe alternative, our findings may be of considerable public health importance", says Tanya Froehlich, MD, a developmental pediatrician at Cincinnati Children's and the study's author.

Pyrethroids were considered a safer choice because they are not as acutely toxic as the banned organophosphates. Animal studies, on the other hand, suggest a heightened vulnerability to the effects of pyrethroid exposure on hyperactivity, impulsivity, and abnormalities in the dopamine system in male mice.

In the newest study, researchers studied data on 687 children 8–15 years of age. Pesticide exposure measurements were collected in a random sample of the urine of half the 8–11 year olds and a third of the 12–15 year olds. Boys with detectable urinary 3-PBA, a biomarker of exposure to pyrethroids, were three times as likely to have ADHD compared with those without detectable 3-PBA. Hyperactivity and impulsivity increased by 50% for every 10-fold increase in 3-PBA levels in boys. Biomarkers were not associated with increased odds of ADHD diagnosis or symptoms in girls.

Gluten intolerance

The connection between celiac disease, psychiatric disorders, and psychological disturbances such as ADHD has been reported repeatedly. Many different mental symptoms and disorders are commonly seen in patients with celiac disease. These include depression, sensory deficit, dyslexia, and anxiety disorders. It has also been found that a significant number of patients with celiac disease suffer from ADHD-like symptoms.

In one study, a gluten-free diet lasting for at least six months significantly improved ADHD symptoms in patients with celiac disease. The results further suggested that celiac disease and gluten intolerance should be considered as a cause of ADHD. Furthermore, there is a close connection between anxiety disorders and celiac disease. In a study, 9 of 15 children with celiac disease with behavioural disturbances were put on a gluten-free diet. Their mood and behavioural disturbances improved.

Technology

Hypnosis is the act of putting people into a trance-like state where they have heightened suggestibility and lose the ability to think critically and logically, which allows easier access to the subconscious mind. In this state, subliminal messages can be easily planted without a person's knowledge. This happens to most people, particularly young children, when they watch television or play video games.

Television causes the brain to slow down, producing a pattern of low-frequency brainwaves and reducing the capacity for higher thought processes. Excessive television viewing by a small child causes the brain to miss some of the early development state, limiting creative ability and higher levels of abstract thinking. Television affects intelligence and attention, and can worsen disorders such as ADHD and contribute to problems such as violence and aggression, personality changes, and underdeveloped social skills.

Television and cell phones are but two examples of our exposure to different EMFs. Add in computers, video games, microwaves, and the various electronics in our modern world, and it doesn't take long to realize we are swimming in an ocean of electromagnetic frequencies. In modern life, this is not about to change. In fact, we will see more and more new developments that increase conveniences but add more electromagnetic stressors to our lives. We can't avoid these modern advances, but we can be aware of the effects of these various frequencies on our mental and physical health and limit our exposures as much as possible.

The book *A Wellness Guide for The Digital Age* by Kerry Crofton, PhD, is an excellent source of additional information that provides sound advice as well as safer solutions for all things wired and wireless.

Autism and genetically modified organisms (GMOs)

Stephanie Seneff, PhD, a head researcher at the Massachusetts Institute of Technology, has studied biology, technology, and nutrition and health for over 30 years. She recently stated: "At today's rate, by 2025, one in two children will be autistic". She noted that the side effects of autism closely mimic those of glyphosate toxicity, and presented data showing a consistent correlation between the use of Roundup on crops and the creation of Roundup-ready genetically modified crop seeds with rising rates of autism. Children with autism have biomarkers indicative of excessive glyphosate, including zinc and iron deficiency, low serum sulphate, seizures, and mitochondrial disorder. (Refer to Chapter 4 for more general information on GMOs.)

Stimulants, Antidepressants, and Brain Development: Misuse and Abuse?

Stimulant medications are the most widely used in the treatment of ADHD. The most commonly used include Adderall, Concerta, Dexedrine, Ritalin, Focalin, Metadate, Cylert, and Vyvanse.

Today, more than 17 million children worldwide have been prescribed psychiatric drugs so dangerous that medicine regulatory agencies in Europe, Australia, and the US have issued warnings about them. For example, antidepressants can cause suicide and hostility in children, adolescents, and young adults up to age 25. The US Food and Drug Administration (FDA) has also issued a warning that stimulant drugs, such as Ritalin and Concerta, can cause suicidal, as well as violent, aggressive, and psychotic behaviour, and that these same drugs can cause heart attacks, stroke, and sudden death.

The National Center for Health Statistics says that 5% of North Americans ages 12–19 years use antidepressants, and another 6% of the same age group use medication (amphetamines) for ADHD. In total, this represents about four million teenagers.

The results of a comprehensive review of pediatric trials conducted between 1988 and 2006, published in 2007 in the *Journal of the American Medical Association,* suggested that the risks of antidepressant medications likely outweigh their benefits to children and adolescents with major depression and anxiety disorders. In response, the FDA adopted a "black box" label warning indicating that antidepressants may increase the risk of suicidal thinking and behaviour in some children and adolescents with depressive disorder. A black box warning is the most serious type of warning in prescription drug labelling.

Amphetamines

The stimulants methylphenidate and amphetamines are mostly prescribed for ADHD. They are Schedule II drugs, meaning they have the same potential for abuse as morphine, opium, and cocaine.

Amphetamine research findings

- A study published in *JAMA Psychiatry* in 1995 investigated the pharmacokinetics of methylphenidate hydrochloride (Ritalin) in the human brain compared with those of cocaine, and evaluated whether cocaine and methylphenidate compete for the same binding sites. The results concluded "because the experience of the 'high' is associated with the fast uptake of cocaine and methylphenidate in the brain, the slow clearance of methylphenidate from the brain may serve as a limiting factor in promoting its frequent administration".

- In 1995, The US Department of Justice stated that "Of particular concern is that ADHD literature prepared for public consumption does not address the potential or actual abuse of methylphenidate. Instead, methylphenidate is routinely portrayed as a benign, mild substance that is not associated with abuse or serious side effects. In reality, however, the scientific literature indicates that methylphenidate shares the same abuse potential as other Schedule II stimulants. Further, case reports document that methylphenidate abuse can lead to tolerance and severe psychological dependence".

- In March 2015, Canada issued warnings about the two main drug classes that are used to treat ADHD – methylphenidate and amphetamine-based drugs. The agency completed safety reviews, and reported stronger and clearer warnings about risks associated with these drugs, including suicidal thoughts and behaviour. The drugs are: Adderall XR, Concerta, Biphentin, Strattera, Intuniv XR, Dexedrine, Ritalin, and Vyvanse.

- A study published in the *British medical Journal*, May 2016 found that methylphenidate increases the risk for arrhythmias by more than 60% overall and that the risk more than triples for individuals with congenital heart disease.

Study investigator Nicole Pratt, PhD, told Medscape Medical News that "parents and clinicians should be aware of the potential for cardiac adverse effects."

Ritalin Abuse

Use of Ritalin (methylphenidate) is a big problem in Canada, especially in the province of British Columbia (BC). The number of prescriptions for medications used to treat ADHD in BC tripled in the past decade, according to the Ministry of Health. At the request of *The Vancouver Sun,* ministry staff checked the province's prescription tracking system, PharmaNet, and found that 312,304 prescriptions to treat ADHD were filled in 2011, while 94,251 were filled in 2000.

With the increase in diagnosis, comes an increase in the use of medications. In 2000, 43% of Canadian children with ADHD were taking medications; in 2007, it was 59%. The study's data come from a sample of Canadian children 3–9 years of age who participated in the National Longitudinal Survey on Children and Youth.

Our penchant for the pills has pegged Canada, after Iceland and the US, as one of the world's top three consumers of methylphenidate, including Ritalin and similar drugs, according to the 2009 Annual Report of the *UN International Narcotic Control Board.* A 2007 US report on the global use of ADHD drugs also singled out Canada for "higher than expected" consumption.

ADHD Drugs Don't Work

A recent study in Quebec looked at medication usage and educational outcomes of nearly 4,000 students in the province over an average of 11 years. Researchers found that boys who took ADHD drugs actually performed worse in school than those with a similar number of symptoms who didn't take the drugs. Girls taking the medicine reported more emotional problems, according to a working paper from the National Bureau of Economic Research, a non-profit economics research firm. The author of the study, Janet Currie, director of the Center for Health and Wellbeing, a health policy institute at Princeton University states "The possibility that (medication) won't help them (in school) needs to be acknowledged and needs to be closely monitored". She also says that side effects and other drawbacks outweigh the benefits.

Given the fact that we don't know a whole lot about how these drugs affect brain development over the long term, why are doctors so quick to put children on them? What's the alternative?

Alternatives to ADHD Drugs

As in any condition, there are times when prescription medications are necessary. When it comes to prescribing stimulants for children with ADHD, it may be necessary in some cases. However, to prescribe a potentially dangerous medication to anyone, but specifically a young child, without a proper diagnosis or knowing the other options available, is unconscionable. Parents are not informed about all the potential risks to their child when they agree to a psychiatric drug prescription.

Millions of children are prescribed these drugs when they have not been properly assessed. Some have simply never been taught to read, or may be suffering from results of a poor diet, allergies, gluten sensitivities, food additive reactions, gut microbiota imbalances, vitamin and mineral deficiencies, brain inflammation, lead poisoning, pesticide exposure, or other environmental toxic effects that can cause various brain disorders. There are many effective and safe treatment options for children and adults who have learning disorders, including ADHD.

Support for People with Learning Disorders

The following general supplements, dietary guidelines, and tips may be of use for people with learning disorders, including ADHD. In the more severe cases such as in autism, more specific assessments and individual supplement treatment programs are required.

Supplement Support for Children with Learning Disorders and ADHD

Review the information in Fundamental Building Blocks of Brain Development section at the beginning of this chapter as a base for nutrient support for optimal brain development in children. For those with learning disorders, additional supplemental and dietary support may be required:

- **Iron** – HemoFactors® is an easily assimilated iron supplement found in health food stores that can be safely taken by children who have confirmed iron deficiency through lab tests of ferritin and hemoglobin, as well as red blood cell count. Do not rely on hemoglobin count alone; ferritin is more important.

- **Zinc** – Children and adults who have ADHD frequently have abnormally low plasma zinc levels, which may interfere with optimal information processing and correlate with the severity of inattentive symptoms. In a large 12-week double-blind placebo-controlled trial, children and adolescents who were randomized to a high dose of zinc (150 mg daily) experienced significant improvement in hyperactivity and impulsivity, but not inattention, over those receiving placebo. In another study, the addition of zinc to methylphenidate therapy resulted in greater improvement than methylphenidate alone.

- **Phosphatidylserine** – This has been clinically proven to provide safe effective treatment in children with ADHD. In the study, 200 ADHD children were randomized to receive either PS/omega-3 or a placebo, and efficacy was assessed using standard rating scales. Analysis of children with a more pronounced hyperactive/impulsive behaviour, as well as mood and behaviour-dysregulation, revealed a significant reduction in the ADHD-index and hyperactive components. Data indicated sustained efficacy for children who continued to receive PS/omega-3. The dosage used in the trial was as follows: Weeks 0–15: 300 mg daily; Weeks 16–30: 150 mg daily.

- **Vitamin C** – Some children may benefit from extra vitamin C or a daily dose of grapeseed or pine bark extracts. One study found that one month of daily supplementation with Pycnogenol (a proprietary pine bark extract) at a dose of 1 mg per kg of body weight improved attention and concentration in children with ADHD. Children between the ages of four and 12 years should get no more than 50% of the adult recommendation for antioxidants, and adolescents and teens should limit their upper intake to those for adults.

- *Bacopa monnieri* – This herb is used in Ayurvedic medicine as a tonic and memory enhancer. A 12-week double-blind randomized trial was conducted in 36 children with ADHD. Those taking bacopa showed significant improvement over those receiving a placebo in tests of sentence repetition, logical memory, and pair-associative learning.

- **Acetyl-L-carnitine** – This compound is required for energy metabolism and synthesis of fatty acids. Findings of a small randomized placebo-controlled study suggest that acetyl-L-carnitine significantly reduces the severity of ADHD symptoms. In a 16-week pilot study, 112 children with ADHD, 5–12 years of age, were randomized to receive placebo or acetyl-L-carnitine. Results showed significant improvement in the acetyl-L-carnitine group over placebo in inattentive-type children. However, there was no improvement over placebo in combined-type ADHD children. Doses of 50 mg/kg daily were used in the study.

- **Deanol** – This acetylcholine precursor has been reported to help with mood and improve memory and learning. Deanol has been used as a treatment for childhood hyperactivity for years. In one study, children were given deanol, methylphenidate, or placebo in a double-blind fashion for three months. Children taking both deanol and methylphenidate showed significant improvement on a number of tests, and researchers concluded that deanol can improve performance in children with learning and behavioural disorders.

- **Pine bark extract** – Pycnogenol, an extract from the bark of the French maritime pine, consisting of phenolic acids, catechin, taxifolin, and procyanidins, is effective for treating ADHD, at least in boys. A study reported in the *European Child & Adolescent Psychiatry* journal in May 2006 found that the pine bark extract group had a significant reduction in hyperactivity and improved attention, visual-motor coordination, and concentration, whereas there were no positive effects noted in the placebo group.

- **EFAs** have been proven effective in the treatment of learning disorders, as mentioned earlier. Look for a supplement containing both EPA and DHA.

- **A children's multivitamin and mineral** is very important to supply the basic nutrients missing from the diet that help support optimal brain development.

Dietary Tips for Children with Learning Disorders and ADHD

Children's behaviour often deteriorates in the late morning and late afternoon, or 3–4 hours after a meal, whether the child has ADHD or not. Children simply run out of fuel. When blood sugar levels go down, stress hormones kick in to raise it up again, but this can cause behavioural problems and diminished concentration. To smooth out the blood sugar mood swings, let children graze on nutritious food throughout the day. Send snacks to school that are high in proteins and good fats for mid-morning and mid-afternoon snacks.

When you are away from home, carry snacks with you to avoid the blood sugar dips and melt downs. While at home, keep a supply of healthy snacks readily available in the pantry or refrigerator. Leave a vegetable tray with the child's favourite dips, cheese cubes, celery or apples spread with peanut butter, hummus, small containers of yogourt, and small containers of raw sunflower, pumpkin, almonds, and cashews, mixed with a few raisins. These are quick nutritious snacks for kids to nibble on throughout the day.

A healthy diet and lifestyle are important for any age and stage of life in order to maintain optimal three brain health. More and more people, both young and old, are being diagnosed with brain disorders, including anxiety, depression, insomnia, learning disorders, and dementias. In Section 4 you will learn about some of the causes and risk factors associated with these conditions, as well as suggestions on how to prevent and treat these life-limiting disorders.

Three-Brain Disorders

Many factors can disrupt the finely tuned three-brain orchestra. When the different players or sections in the orchestra are not "in sync", this desynchronized rhythm can cause many different mental and emotional symptoms, as well as brain disorders.

Mood Disorders

Mood disorders affect about 15% of the population in Canada. Everyone experiences cycles of emotional ups and downs, however people with mood disorders experience them with greater intensity and for longer periods of time than most people.

Depression is the most common mood disorder, and anxiety disorder is the most common mental health problem in Canada. It is sad but true: people under 20 years of age have the highest rate of depression, while those 20–29 years of age have the highest rate of anxiety symptoms. Suicide accounts for 24% of all deaths among Canadians 15–24 years of age and 16% in those age 25–44. The World Health Organization lists depression as one of the leading causes of disability worldwide.

Nutrients and Mental Health Problems

One thing the conventional medical community may agree on, at least for the most part, is that neurotransmitters have an influence on mental health disorders and behaviour, and that this is genetically determined. However, what is not agreed upon is the role of nutrients like vitamins and minerals.

Neurotransmitter problems, in some cases, have a genetic component that involves absorption, metabolism, or storage of key nutrients, and some people benefit from medications. However, for many people, medications have too many negative side effects and/or they are ineffective. Moreover, the underlying cause of the mental health problem still remains. Nutrient therapy, diet, and lifestyle, along with addressing any other factors such as microbiota imbalances in the gut brain, food allergies, inflammation, and blood sugar imbalances, can be a very potent and effective treatment for many people with brain disorders, without the risk of side effects. (Refer to Chapters 3 and 4 for more information on "brain busters" that can contribute to different mental health problems.)

The Pfeiffer Treatment Center has amassed a large database of biochemical information from more than 10,000 patients with mental health problems. Examination of this data shows that most of these persons have striking abnormalities in specific nutrients required for neurotransmitter production.

According to the *Diagnostic and Statistical Manual of Mental Disorders,* depression, bipolar disorder, schizophrenia, and obsessive compulsive disorders (OCD) are among the most common mental disorders. Incidence rates vary, from 26% in North America to 4% in China. Some of this difference may be due to how mental health disorders are diagnosed. However, it can also be explained by study findings indicating that a lack of certain dietary nutrients, namely essential vitamins, minerals, and omega-3 fatty acids, contribute to the development of mental disorders. These nutrients are often deficient in the general population in North America, as well as in other developed countries, and are shown to be exceptionally deficient in patients suffering from mental health disorders.

Supplements that contain amino acids are converted to specific neurotransmitters that can alleviate symptoms of many mental health disorders caused by problems in one or more of the three brains. More recent scientific evidence has shown that nutritional supplementation has proven beneficial in helping to control symptoms of major depression, bipolar disorder, schizophrenia, anxiety disorders, eating disorders, attention deficit disorder/attention deficit hyperactivity disorder (ADD/ADHD), addiction, and autism. In addition to supporting disorders in the head brain, nutritional supplements have been proven to be effective in supporting disorders of the gut and heart brains as well.

The first step is a proper medical diagnosis that includes an outline of all the possible treatment options available to the individual. The final decision on whether or not to try nutritional supplements as a treatment must be the decision of the patient. New clinical studies are being published daily on the positive effects of nutritional and supplement therapies on all types of disorders and diseases, and although it may take time for health care practitioners to become educated and aware of the options available, this option should not be ignored.

Diagnosing Depression

It is normal to feel down or out of sorts some of the time. You may also have wondered if you are depressed. There are several types of depressive episodes that can last months, or sometimes years, and can interfere with all aspects of life, such as social interactions and work functioning.

According to the *Diagnostic and Statistical Manual of Mental Disorders*, to be considered depressed, you need to have at least five of the following symptoms:

- Depressed mood most of the day, nearly every day
- Markedly diminished interest or pleasure in all, or almost all activities
- Significant weight loss when not dieting or weight gain, or decrease or increase in appetite
- Insomnia or sleeping too much nearly every day
- Psychomotor agitation (unintentional motion caused from muscle tension)
- Fatigue or loss of energy almost daily
- Feeling of worthlessness, or excessive or inappropriate guilt
- Diminished ability to think or concentrate or indecisiveness
- Recurrent thoughts of death, suicidal thoughts or attempt

However, whether you "fit" the depression diagnosis is not the most important thing. If you are feeling so down that you feel you need to do something about it, then that is the most important factor.

Brain imbalances that cause anxiety and mood disorders such as depression are most often related to other factors that are seldom addressed in Western medicine. It is important to treat the cause of any condition. For example:

- Many people are diagnosed with depression when they really are not depressed, they are simply exhausted and do not have the energy for life. It is very common for people who are diagnosed with depression and anxiety to have adrenal fatigue and/or thyroid disorders. The adrenal glands are the main stress adaptive organs. Chronic stress can cause adrenal fatigue, resulting in many symptoms similar to the classic depression diagnosis criteria. Symptoms such as low energy, sleep problems, mood swings, depression, anxiety, and weight loss or weight gain are common in people with adrenal fatigue. Most cases of anxiety have underlying adrenal dysregulation.

- Symptoms of thyroid disorders include anxiety, emotional volatility, irritability, lack of focus and attention, depression, insomnia, changes in appetite, loss of interest and initiative, and poor memory. If left untreated, thyroid disorders are commonly misdiagnosed as dementia.

- Gut brain problems such as microbiota imbalance can also cause symptoms of depression. Evidence shows that bowel disorders are often correlated with poor mood. In fact, 20% of patients with functional bowel disorders such as irritable bowel syndrome (IBS) have a diagnosable psychiatric illness. Almost one-third of patients with IBS have been found to have anxiety or depression. (Refer to Chapter 5 for a more detailed discussion of the gut-brain connection.)

- Canadian researchers found that a protein known to be a marker of inflammation was up to one-third higher in the brains of depressed patients compared to healthy ones. Those with the most severe forms of depression also had the most inflammation.

- Inflammation is the cause of depression in many people. If people with depression fail to respond after two trials of antidepressants, they are considered treatment resistant. Perhaps a better term might be "incorrectly diagnosed". Cytokines are associated with treatment-resistant depression. They actually tend to decrease the function of serotonin. Serotonin is one of the neurotransmitters often associated with depression, are probably not the cause of depression. In one study, treatment-resistant patients taking antidepressants were supplemented with the addition of aspirin, an anti-inflammatory agent. More than 50% of these patients responded to this combined treatment, and at the end of the study more than 80% of the group responsive to the anti-inflammatory agent went into remission.

- The heart brain and depression are closely connected. Depression is commonly present in patients with coronary heart disease (CHD) and is independently associated with increased cardiovascular morbidity and mortality. In comparison with nondepressed individuals, depressed patients with CHD frequently have higher levels of biomarkers found to predict cardiac events or promote atherosclerosis.

- Studies show that elevated levels of C-reactive protein are not only associated with increased risk for cardiovascular diseases, but also with increased risk for psychological distress and depression in the general population.

- Sugar consumption has been linked to depression, anxiety, suicide, irritability, anger outbursts, anxiety, fatigue, and lethargy. Sugar is a "mood-altering drug".

- Hypoglycemia (low blood sugar) has a profound effect on moods.

- Vitamin D deficiency has been repeatedly observed in conditions involving inflammation, such as cardiovascular disease, diabetes, anxiety, and depression. New research shows that low serum levels of vitamin D are associated with clinically significant symptoms of depression in otherwise healthy individuals.

- Other causes of anxiety and mood disorders include environmental toxins and heavy metals, hormonal imbalances, and food allergies and intolerances.

Depression in Teens

A survey released by the World Health Organization (WHO) in May 2014 found depression to be the number one cause of illness and disability in adolescents worldwide. The reasons for this increase are uncertain, but we know there is an association between stress and depression. A new survey from the American Psychological Association in 2014 reported that teen stress rivals that of adults.

The World Mental Health Survey found that half of those who suffered from mental health problems, including depression, first experience symptoms at the age of 14. Only half of adolescents with a mental health problem receive treatment. In North America today, high school and university/college students are 5–8 times as likely to suffer from depressive symptoms compared with teenagers 50 or 60 years ago.

Some experts suggest it is because children are more exposed to stress, which has significant implications for how a child develops and can increase vulnerability for anxiety and depression; others suggest the role of family and media. A study from the National Institutes of Health found that media portrayals of body image and the "ideal" life create unrealistic expectations for teenagers, disrupting their "normal identity development", thus leading to depression.

Men and Depression

It is estimated that 11% of Canadian men are diagnosed with depression each year. However, the percentage is probably much higher considering that most men will not seek help for depression and other related disorders such as anxiety, mood disorders, or insomnia. The long-term consequences of masked depression can be devastating and too many men are suffering. The likelihood that women will develop depression in their lifetime is twice as likely as men. However women are more likely to seek help. So why do men resist seeking support for personal health problems?

Even in this time of gender equality and mixing of stereotypical roles and traits in North America, masculinity is still associated with physical strength, emotional stoicism, assertiveness, and control. So if men admit to what is perceived as a weakness such as illness or injury, they feel they do not conform to this idealized masculinity. At an early age, boys learn to "take it like a man" because showing vulnerability or weakness poses a threat to stereotypical masculinity.

Beliefs about masculinity not only affect a man's general lack of interest in health issues; many men simply don't believe they are susceptible to depression or other mental health disorders and hold the attitude "real men don't get depression". Rather than seeking help, it is common for men to try to mask their depression, and it is often expressed through behaviour such as verbal abusiveness or aggression, hostility, irritability, or drinking to excess.

Overview of Antidepressant Medications

The scope of this book does not allow for an in-depth discussion about the various medications available to treat depression. However, a brief explanation may shed some light on why some medications seem to work for some people, while other medications do not.

More than 160 million antidepressant prescriptions are written annually, despite the fact that a recent meta-analysis showed they are no more effective than placebo to treat mild-to-moderate depression, the most common condition for which they are prescribed. Other studies have revealed that these medications can cause a host of problems, including sexual adverse effects, infertility, increased risk of weight gain and diabetes, blood pressure problems, cardiac deaths, heart defects in unborn children, and even suicide. However, antidepressant medications are effective in severe cases and should be considered as first-line therapy in those patients.

Medications used to treat depression work in different ways. The tricyclic antidepressants, such as imipramine, work by regulating the limbic-hypothalamic-pituitary-adrenal (LHPA) axis in the hippocampus and brain cortex. On the other hand, selective serotonin reuptake inhibitors (SSRIs) such as fluoxetine (Prozac) are unable to prevent stress-induced elevation in cortisol and overactivity of the LHPA axis.

Some clinical studies have found that the tricyclic antidepressants are more effective than the SSRIs in the treatment of melancholia, a severe form of depression characterized by complete loss of the capacity for pleasure. Patients with melancholia also tend to have high cortisol levels. For these patients and those with both depression and anxiety, it was found that Effexor, an antidepressant with both norepinephrine and 5-HTP reuptake activity, was reported to be more effective than Prozac. It is very hard to know which antidepressant is going to be effective, and it often requires a process of trial and error. One simple test that could be done to help determine what medication to try is a salivary or blood cortisol level test. This simple example may explain why some people don't respond to antidepressant medications.

Supplement Support for Depression

"Hey, you know, breakdowns come and breakdowns go. So what are you going to do about it? That's what I'd like to know."– Paul Simon, Gumboots

Several natural supplements have proven effective in the treatment of mild-to-moderate depression.

5-hydroxytryptophan

Depression and anxiety have been linked to serotonin imbalances in the brain. 5-hydroxytryptophan (5-HTP) is a building block for serotonin and it also increases endorphin levels (the feel-good brain chemicals). Numerous studies have shown that 5-HTP is as effective as SSRIs and tricyclic antidepressants, with fewer side effects.

Dosage: 100–200 mg 2–3 times daily.

Saffron (*Crocus sativus* L. stigma)

Saffron has been shown to be an effective natural antidepressant in several clinical trials. One study compared the effects of saffron with fluoxetine (generic form of Prozac). Both treatments resulted in significant improvements in depression symptoms and severity, with no difference in the amount of improvement between the two groups. Saffron's antidepressant properties seem to be related to serotonin metabolism. In another study, saffron was compared to the tricyclic antidepressant imipramine. The effects were found comparable in the treatment of mild-to-moderate depression without the common side effects of imipramine such as dry mouth and sedation.

Dosage: 30 mg daily.

Inositol

Meta-analysis results suggest that inositol has beneficial effects in mental health disorders, including mood disorders like depression, bipolar depression, and panic.

Dosage: 400–4000 mg daily, depending on the individual.

Vitamin B6 (pyridoxal 5-phosphate)

Vitamin B6 is required as a coenzyme for the biosynthesis of several neurotransmitters, including gamma-aminobutyric acid (GABA), dopamine, norepinephrine, and serotonin. Vitamin B6 concentrations in the brain are about 100 times higher than levels in the blood, so it is not surprising that vitamin B6 deficiency has neurological effects including depression, insomnia, and mental confusion.

Dosage: 50–100 mg daily.

LOOK for a product such as…

Cloud Nine, that contains important nutrients including inositol, saffron, 5-hydroxytryptophan, and vitamin B6.

Curcumin

Curcumin plays a significant role in the treatment of inflammatory brain conditions such as depression, dementias including Alzheimer's disease, and symptoms related to traumatic brain injuries. Curcumin has also been proven beneficial in the treatment of stress-induced behavioural, memory, and learning problems. Curcumin supports the three brains. (Refer to Chapters 3 on inflammation and Chapter 9 on memory disorders, for more information on the benefits of curcumin.)

Dosage: 300 mg daily of a brand that has been optimized for maximum absorption.

Omega-3 fatty acids

Depression and anxiety appear to be linked to lower levels of omega-3 fatty acids. Both depression and anxiety can enhance the production of pro-inflammatory compounds known as cytokines, and omega-3 fatty acids found in fish oils and flax oils decrease this elevation. Psychological stress can also cause an elevation of these cytokines. Studies suggest that the anti-inflammatory role of omega-3 fatty acids may influence brain-derived neurotrophic factor (BDNF) in depression. BDNF has been found to be negatively correlated with the severity of depressive symptoms. Omega-3 fatty acids support the three brains.

Dosage: 1000–3000 mg daily.

Probiotics

New research shows that gut bacteria communicate with and influence head brain function. An imbalance in the good and bad gut microbiota, called dysbiosis, is associated with a number of brain disorders and symptoms. These include ADHD, autism, OCD, mood swings, memory problems, anxiety, depression, and insomnia. Probiotics support the three brains. A combination of *Bifidobacterium longum* and *Lactobacillus helveticus* have proven beneficial for stress-related mental health disorders. (Refer to Chapter 1 for more information on the gut microbiota and probiotics.)

Dosage: depends on the product. Follow the manufacturer's directions.

St. John's wort *(Hypericum perforatum)*

St. John's wort has been used in traditional medicine for centuries to treat a wide range of disorders and is licensed in Germany to treat anxiety, depression, and sleep disorders. It was proven as effective as standard antidepressants in many clinical trials for the treatment of mild to moderate depression. It also has fewer side effects.

Dosage: 300 mg 1–3 times daily, standardized to 0.3% hypericin.

Phosphatidylserine

Phosphatidylserine (PS) can offset the body's response to physical stress by decreasing the level of stress hormones. Researchers have also found that PS reduces anxiety and helps alleviate stress-induced depression. PS (300 mg daily) was given to depressed geriatric patients not exhibiting dementia. Researchers noted significant improvement in depressive symptoms after 30 days. Memory and behavioural symptoms were also improved compared to placebo.

Dosage: 100–300 mg daily.

 LOOK for a product such as...

Rather than purchasing each of the above-mentioned products individually, some brands offer a comprehensive "kit" that includes the most essential supplements for brain health in convenient daily packets. For example, **Daily Brain** includes phosphatidylserine-enriched sunflower (containing naturally occurring phosphatidylcholine [PC], phosphatidylinositol [PI], and phosphatidylethanolamine [PE]), curcumin, omega-3 fatty acids EPA and DHA, grapeseed extract, and key probiotic strains.

LOOK for a product such as...

Brain Defence, that combines important anti-inflammatory and cognitive support such as bacopa, ashwagandha, curcumin, boswellia, and chamomile. (Refer to Chapter 3 for more information and research on inflammation and disorders of the three brains.)

Berries for the Brain

Recent research has shown that New Zealand blackcurrants help keep the brain mentally young and agile. This finding could have potential in managing the mental decline associated with aging populations, or in helping people with brain disorders such as Parkinson's disease or depression.

Participants in the study, 36 healthy adults 18–35 years of age, consumed a 250 mL (9 oz) drink prior to conducting a set of demanding mental performance assessments. The participants consumed either a placebo, or an anthocyanin-rich drink made from berries, or a cold-pressed juice made from New Zealand blackcurrants. The assessments showed that attention and mood were improved in the groups consuming the anthocyanin-rich drink and the blackcurrant drink, and mental fatigue was reduced. In addition, blood tests showed that the activity of the monoamine oxidase enzymes (MAOs) was strongly decreased. MAOs regulate serotonin and dopamine concentrations in the brain. These chemicals are known to affect mood and cognition, and are the focus for treatments of both the neurodegenerative symptoms associated with Parkinson's and mood disorders.

This study strongly supports the potential for antioxidant compounds found in blackcurrants and other berries to support three-brain health.

Anxiety Disorders

The National Institute of Mental Health reports that by 2020, anxiety-related disorders will affect 7 out of 10 individuals in North America alone. Even in developing countries, where four-fifths of world's people live, the next decade will bring a dramatic change as anxiety-oriented disorders replace the traditional enemies such as infection.

What Are Anxiety Disorders?

Like many other mental health conditions, anxiety disorders seem to be a result of a combination of biological, psychological, genetic, and other individual factors.

The neurotransmitters (chemical messengers) in the brain involved in anxiety include serotonin, norepinephrine, and GABA. In many cases, these neurotransmitter imbalances are caused by acute or chronic stress. Certain medical conditions, such as stress-induced adrenal fatigue, anemia, and thyroid problems, can also cause symptoms of anxiety.

The most common anxiety disorders include OCD, post-traumatic stress disorder (PTSD), social anxiety disorder, and general anxiety disorders. These are collectively the most common mental health disorders in North America. Each anxiety disorder has different symptoms, but all of the symptoms cluster around excessive, irrational fear and dread that compromise a person's life to one degree or another.

General symptoms of anxiety include excessive worry about little things, increased startle reflex, fear of crowds, jumpiness, impaired concentration, ongoing irrational thoughts, restless sleep or insomnia, muscle tension, and irritability or edginess. Panic attacks include symptoms such as palpitations, pounding or rapid heart rate, sweating and body temperature changes, trembling, shortness of breath, chest pain and discomfort, nausea or digestive distress, dizziness and light-headedness, and fear of losing control or "going crazy".

Stress Hormones and Anxiety Disorders

Along with glucocorticoids, the adrenal glands secrete another class of hormones called catecholamines. Norepinephrine (NE) and epinephrine (E) are the main catecholamines often associated with the fight-or-flight response in acute stress. NE can increase heart rate and blood pressure, as well as create a sense of overwhelming fear. Low levels of NE are associated with loss of alertness or motivation, poor memory, ADHD, and depression. Most anxiety symptoms are due to elevated NE levels.

The fight-or-flight response is a chemical reaction to a real or perceived life-threatening situation. Excess amounts of NE and E are produced, which provide extra strength and energy needed to run or to fight. This reaction is needed for survival reactions like running from a bear in the woods. However, when these hormones become elevated during normal activity, they cause anxiety, and sudden increases cause full-blown panic attacks. Cortisol and other stress hormones increase the permeability of the blood-brain barrier, a protective barrier that prevents toxic substances from entering the brain. As a result of the increased permeability, more chemicals and toxins can enter the brain, many of which are excitotoxins that cause overstimulation of the brain, causing anxiety.

The Gut-Brain Axis: How the Microbiome Influences Anxiety and Depression

The human intestine harbours nearly 100 trillion bacteria that are essential for health. Based on recent discoveries, gut microbiota play a significant role in how the gut and head brains communicate. They also influence the risk of disease and mental health disorders, including anxiety and depression.

Stress influences the composition of the gut microbiota, and the gut microbiota affects the stress reactivity of the hypothalamic-pituitary-adrenal (HPA) axis. Depressive episodes are associated with dysregulation of the HPA axis, and stress-induced changes in the microbiota also increase inflammation, contributing to depression, dementias, and other brain disorders.

Stress is known to increase intestinal permeability, causing a leaky gut. This allows pathogens the opportunity to cross the gut barrier and directly affect immune cells and neurons of the gut brain. A recent study has shown that pretreating rodents with the probiotic lactobacillus reduced the intestinal permeability typically resulting from stress and also prevented associated HPA hyper-reactivity.

Although the use of probiotics in animal studies has consistently shown an impact on anxiety and depressive behaviours, there is limited work published on the effects of probiotics on depression or anxiety symptoms in humans. The studies that do exist provide evidence that probiotics have similar antidepressive and anti-anxiety effects in humans:

- In a double-blind, placebo-controlled clinical trial, healthy subjects were given a mixture of probiotics containing lactobacillus and bifidus or placebo for 30 days. The probiotic treatment group demonstrated significantly less psychological distress than did matched controls.

- In another double-blind, placebo-controlled trial, healthy subjects were fed either a probiotic-containing milk drink or placebo control for three weeks. Mood and cognition were assessed before treatment and after 10 and 20 days of consumption. Subjects who initially scored in the lowest third for depressed mood showed significant improvement in symptoms after probiotic treatment.

- Chronic fatigue syndrome (CFS) is a disorder caused by chronic stress that is frequently associated with fatigue, insomnia, anxiety, and gastrointestinal disturbance. In a pilot study, patients with CFS receiving lactobacillus daily for two months showed significantly fewer anxiety symptoms than did the placebo group.

Although these clinical studies examining the impact of probiotics on mood and anxiety are in the early stages, the results are promising. Targeting microbiota and the gut-brain axis seems to have effective and safe therapeutic potential in mood and anxiety disorders.

In general, people are looking for safe and effective treatments for their anxieties, tension, stress, and insomnia, and they are starting to turn to nonpharmaceuticals such as herbal products and other alternative remedies. Many safe options are available that can effectively treat people with depression, anxiety, and other brain disorders. Remember, it is most important to address an important underlying cause: the adrenal stress and stressors.

Supplement Support for Anxiety Disorders

Most anxiety disorders are due to elevated stress hormones. Chapter 2 provided suggestions to help keep the nervous system calm and prevent the overproduction of stress hormones. In addition to stress support, other herbs and vitamins have been found to be effective in the treatment of anxiety.

GABA

GABA is the most important inhibitory neurotransmitter in the brain. It acts like a brake in times of increased stress, eliciting a sense of calm. Low levels of GABA have been linked to anxiety, depression, and insomnia. GABA increases the production of alpha brainwaves characterized with being relaxed. It also increases mental focus and alertness and reduces beta waves associated with nervousness and hyperactivity. In addition, GABA has been shown to produce relaxation by reducing stress markers such as heart rate, cortisol levels, and pupil diameter.

Dosage: 100–200 mg 2–3 times daily. As a general guideline, it is recommended to take no more than 3000 mg within a 24-hour period.

Magnesium

Magnesium has been found to be effective for the treatment of depression and anxiety. Insomnia, short-term memory loss, irritability, agitation, and headaches are other conditions that may benefit from magnesium supplementation.

Dosage: 400–800 mg daily.

L-theanine

Most of L-theanine's effects have to do with promoting relaxation. It has been shown to stimulate the brain's alpha waves, a state often related to meditation, suggesting that it has the ability to put users into a more relaxed mood. It also reduces beta waves, which are associated with hyperactivity, nervousness, and scattered mind chatter. Studies have shown that L-theanine reduces stress, helps with sleep, and increases mental alertness.

Dosage: 100–200 mg 1–3 times daily.

Kava kava *(Piper methysticum)*

Many cultures have used kava for centuries to relieve anxiety, restlessness, and insomnia. Kava has anti-anxiety effects without sedative or mentally impairing side effects commonly caused by benzodiazepines or antidepressants. Kava can be used for those people tapering off of benzodiazepines.

Dosage: 250 mg 1–2 times daily of an extract standardized to 30% kavalactones.

Passion flower *(Passiflora incarata)*

Passion flower is known as a "calming" herb for anxiety or nervousness, insomnia, generalized anxiety disorder (GAD), ADHD, and palpitations. Recent studies have found passionflower to be comparable to benzodiazepine drugs (e.g., Ativan) in the treatment of anxiety and insomnia, but passionflower resulted in less drowsiness.

Dosage: 2000–4000 mg daily.

Probiotics and prebiotics

Studies show that the probiotics *Bifidobacterium longum* and *Lactobacillus helveticus* have a marked effect on GABA levels, lowering the stress-induced cortisol and resulting in reduced levels of anxiety and depressive behaviour.

Dosage: depends on the type of probiotic or combined probiotic/prebiotic. Follow the manufacturer's instructions.

Omega-3 fatty acids

Depression and anxiety appear to be linked to lower levels of omega-3 fatty acids. Both depression and anxiety can enhance the production of pro-inflammatory compounds known as cytokines. Omega-3 fatty acids found in fish oils and flaxseed oils decrease this elevation in cytokine production. Brain cells require omega-3 to transmit signals that enable proper thinking, moods, and emotions. However, omega-3 oils are often present at very low levels in most North Americans and bipolar sufferers. Numerous clinical trials show that daily intake of omega-3 fatty acids decreases manic/depressive symptoms better than placebo.

Dosage: 1000–3000 mg daily.

Phospholipids and EFAs

Impaired fatty acid and phospholipid metabolism may be a primary cause of depression and bipolar disorders. EFA supplementation is shown to be effective in treating schizophrenia and bipolar disorder, and should also be considered for OCD. A number of epidemiological studies show a significant negative correlation between fish consumption and rates of depression, as well as postpartum depression, bipolar disorder, and seasonal affective disorder (SAD).

Dosage: 200–600 mg daily.

 LOOK for a product such as...

Brilliant Mind, that contains omega-3 fatty acids, phosphatidylcholine (PC), phosphatidylserine (PS), and Alpha-GPC, along with a good antioxidant such as green tea. (Refer to Chapter 5 for more information on phospholipids and EFAs.)

Mood Swings Due to Hypoglycemia

People love their carbohydrates, especially the refined variety, and as a result blood sugar dysregulation is very common in our society. Hypoglycemia occurs when blood glucose (blood sugar) falls to abnormally low levels due to imbalances in the hormones that regulate blood sugar. Glucose is the main fuel for the brain and is required by all cells of the body, therefore it is important to maintain balanced blood glucose levels adequate for meeting the high energy demands of the brain.

After eating, the pancreas releases insulin to move the glucose in the blood into the cells, and thus lowers the blood sugar level. Insulin is responsible for bringing excess blood glucose levels back to normal. If glucose levels drop, the pancreas secretes another hormone called glucagon, triggering the breakdown of stored glycogen in the liver into glucose, which is then released into the bloodstream, bringing glucose levels back up.

However, overabundance of refined carbohydrates and sugars causes the pancreas to overwork, constantly pumping out insulin and glucagon is unable to regulate the effect of the increasing insulin. As a result, blood sugar levels swing from too high to too low rapidly, and this rollercoaster can cause many mental and emotional symptoms.

The mental and emotional symptoms of hypoglycemia include fatigue, rapid mood changes, difficulty concentrating, crying spells, irritability, restlessness, violent outbursts, forgetfulness, anxiety, insomnia, night terrors, temperamental outbursts, depression, and panic attacks. (Refer to Chapter 5 for more information on the effects of insulin on the brain.) Imbalances in the gut microbiota (dysbiosis) can also have a profound effect on blood sugar regulation. (Refer to Chapter 2 for more information on dysbiosis.)

Suggestions for Treatment of Hypoglycemia

- Limit foods with high sugar content, especially on an empty stomach.
- Eliminate or keep to a very minimum, all refined carbohydrates – this includes white breads, pastries, cookies, cakes, pizza, pop, desserts, and all forms of refined sugars including sucrose, fructose, raw sugar, brown sugar, corn syrup, molasses, malt, malted barley, fruit juices, maple syrup, and honey. Refer to glycemic index sources and keep 80–90% of food intake in the low-to-moderate range of the glycemic index. (Refer to Chapter 5 for more information on the glycemic index.)
- Eat small frequent meals and snacks high in protein and fat, as well as a moderate intake of complex carbohydrates. Complex carbohydrates provide the necessary glucose in a slow, gradual manner, and can be thought of as "time-released" sugar for the brain.
- Carry juice or dried fruit for a quick recovery when you feel your blood sugar drop.

- Eat a diet high in fibre, fresh vegetables and fruit, good quality protein, and good oils such as flax and olive – the Mediterranean diet. (Refer to Chapter 5 for more information on the Mediterranean diet.)

Supplement Support for Blood Sugar Imbalances

Chromium picolinate

Chromium supplementation has been shown to alleviate hypoglycemic symptoms and significantly raise serum glucose values. Insulin binding to red blood cells and the number of insulin receptors also improved significantly during chromium supplementation.

Dosage: 200–400 mcg daily.

B vitamins

B vitamins are depleted in times of stress. A deficiency in B6 in particular can contribute to blood sugar problems.

Dosage: 1–2 capsules daily of a B complex or as directed.

PGX®

The health benefits linked to soluble dietary fibre, including stabilizing blood sugar levels, are significantly magnified with PGX. (Refer to Chapter 5 for more information on PGX.)

Dosage: 750–1500 mg before each meal.

 LOOK for a product such as…

For stress support, look for a product such as **Stress Less** containing adaptogenic herbs such as ashwagandha, *Panax ginseng,* and rhodiola, as well as choline and an antioxidant like green tea extract. (Refer to Chapter 2 for more information on stress and adrenal support.)

In addition to the supplement support mentioned above, review the section on cravings later in this chapter.

For many people, following a healthy high-fibre diet low in refined carbohydrates and sugars, along with exercise, may be all that is required to help control glucose levels. For others, this may not be enough, and supplements may need to be taken to sustain glucose in a normal range.

Bipolar Disorder/Manic Depression

Bipolar disorder, also known as manic depression, is a brain disorder that causes unusual shifts in mood, energy, activity levels, and the ability to carry out day-to-day tasks. Everyone goes through ups and downs from time to time, but bipolar symptoms are severe to the point that they can interfere dramatically in a person's life. People with bipolar disorder experience intense emotional states that occur in distinct periods called mood episodes. An overly joyful or overexcited state is called a manic episode, while an extremely sad state is called a depressive episode. Sometimes both occur in a mood episode.

Bipolar disorder usually begins in early adulthood, with the average age of onset around 18–24 years, although it can sometimes start in childhood or as late as the forties or fifties. Research shows that genes play a role – some people with the disorder are more susceptible to emotional and physical stress, which can trigger a manic or depressive episode.

Thanks to an emerging science called epigenetics, researchers have learned that DNA is no longer destiny, and that each of us has the ability to influence how our genes express themselves. With healthy lifestyle choices and environmental changes, the right diet, and nutritional supplements, we can actually alter our gene expression. Some biochemical abnormalities in people with bipolar disorder include excess acetylcholine receptors (which can cause mania and depression), vitamin B deficiencies, taurine deficiency, omega-3 fatty acids deficiencies, and antioxidant deficiency. If a person is already on a mood roller coaster, refined sugar will cause further chaos. Processed refined sugar sends insulin levels soaring, which in turn sparks a craving for more sweet foods. After the sugar fix, a crash follows.

Lithium and Bipolar Disorder

Lithium carbonate has commonly been used in the treatment of bipolar disorders, but high doses are required, which often cause adverse side effects. Another form of lithium, called lithium orotate, is preferred as it more readily crosses the blood-brain barrier and therefore can be used in much lower doses (e.g., 5 mg) with remarkable results and no side effects. In addition, lithium orotate is available without a prescription in the US or from a health care practitioner in Canada (or, in British Columbia, from a naturopathic doctor).

Medications such as lithium, anticonvulsants, antidepressants, and benzodiazepines are commonly prescribed for people with bipolar disorder. Investigating possible causes, whether it is food allergy, heavy metals, stress, etc., and treating accordingly, can effectively help many people with bipolar disorder lead full, productive lives.

Supplement Support for Bipolar Disorder

L-taurine

L-taurine is an amino acid that acts as an inhibitory neurotransmitter, eliciting a calming effect. Its basic function is to help facilitate the movement of sodium, potassium, calcium, and magnesium ions in and out of cells. These minerals are very important in the treatment of mood disorders and specifically bipolar disorder. A deficiency of this amino acid may increase a bipolar patient's manic episodes. Taurine has also been effective in the treatment of migraines, insomnia, restlessness, depression, and irritability.

Dosage: 300–600 mg daily.

L-tyrosine

L-tyrosine is an amino acid that is a precursor to the neurotransmitters dopamine and norepinephrine, as well as the thyroid hormone thyroxin. One theory of depression etiology is that it is based on a deficiency or malfunction of norepinephrine in the brain. The synthesis of these neurotransmitters is affected in chronic stress. Several clinical trials have demonstrated that tyrosine administration reduces effects of stress, including hypertension. Improvements were noted in mood and mental states (happiness, mental clarity, hostility, and tension) as well as cognitive tests. L-tyrosine is excitatory so it should be taken in the morning so it does not interfere with sleep.

Dosage: 800–1200 mg daily.

GABA

GABA is the most important inhibitory neurotransmitter in the brain. It acts like a brake in times of increased stress, eliciting a sense of calm. Low levels of GABA have been linked to anxiety, depression, and insomnia. GABA increases the production of alpha brainwaves characterized by relaxation and greater mental focus and alertness, and reduces beta waves associated with nervousness and hyperactivity. In addition, it has been shown to produce relaxation thorough reducing stress markers such as heart rate, cortisol levels, and pupil diameter.

Dosage: 100–200 mg 2–3 times daily. As a general guideline, it is recommended to take no more than 3000 mg within a 24-hour period.

Magnesium

Magnesium has been found to function similarly to lithium, which is often prescribed for bipolar disorder as a mood stabilizer. Adding magnesium to your diet may help decrease the symptoms of mania or rapid cycling.

Dosage: 400–800 mg daily.

B vitamins (B6, B12, and folic acid)

B6, B12, and folic acid are often low in people with anxiety and depression. Many studies have shown a vitamin B12 deficiency in people diagnosed with bipolar disorder. Since 1984, studies have shown that vitamin B12 supplementation resolves symptoms significantly in people with bipolar disorder.

Dosage: B6: 50–100 mg daily; B12: 1000 mcg of methylcobalamin daily; folic acid: 1–2 mg daily.

Essential fatty acids

Essential fatty acids (EFAs), particularly eicosapentaenoic acid (EPA) and docosahexaenoic acid (DHA), are very important as part of a supplement program for people with mood disorders. (See Chapter 5 for more information on EFAs.)

Dosage: 1000–3000 mg daily of omega-3 fatty acids containing both DHA and EPA.

In addition, the American Psychiatric treatment recommendations for bipolar disorder include the following:

- All adults should eat fish at least twice a week.

- Patients with mood impulse control or psychotic disorders should consume a minimum of 1 g of EPA and DHA daily.

- An omega-3 supplement may be useful in patients with mood disorders (1–9 g daily). Use of more than 3 g daily should be monitored by a health care practitioner.

Food Cravings

As mentioned previously, an imbalance in different neurotransmitters can cause a wide range of neurological symptoms, including relentless overeating and cravings. Mood disorders and food cravings often go hand in hand and are made worse with stress and the increased release of stress hormones. When cortisol and other stress hormones rise, many people crave sugary, fatty, and salty food combinations to "feed" the pleasure and reward circuit governed primarily by the neurotransmitter dopamine, as well as serotonin, GABA, and norepinephrine, to some degree.

Our brains are wired to make us seek out pleasure. When we eat sugary or salty foods, it stimulates the release of dopamine in our brain, which makes us feel pleasure. Our brain recognizes this feeling and likes it, and begins to crave more, resulting in increased dependence on these foods for natural mood elevation. However, the more they are used, the more depleted the natural mood-enhancing brain chemistry becomes.

Some people experience powerful cravings for sweets – internal messages telling them to eat sugar even though they know it is bad for them – and they are unable to control the cravings. It becomes an addiction for some people because when they ingest sugar it makes them feel good for a short period of time, and when they don't have it, they don't feel well. It is interesting to note that sugar binging releases the neurotransmitter dopamine, as do drugs of abuse such as heroin and cocaine. In one study, researchers noted that the symptoms of withdrawal from sugar are similar to withdrawal from morphine or nicotine.

The Gut Brain and Cravings

As previously mentioned, dopamine is known as the feel-good molecule associated with the pleasure and the reward system. It acts the same way in the gut as well, and it is involved in preventing depression and regulating sleep, appetite and cravings, and body temperature.

Such gut brain to head brain signals may also explain why fatty foods make us feel good. When ingested, fatty acids are detected by cell receptors in the lining of the gut, which send nerve signals to the brain. For example, research shows that brain scans of volunteers given fatty acids directly into the gut had a lower response to pictures and music designed to make them feel sad compared to those given saline. They also reported feeling only about half as sad as the other group.

Supplement Support for Cravings

L-glutamine

L-glutamine reaches the starving brain within minutes and can often immediately put a stop to even the most powerful sweet and starch cravings. The brain is fuelled by L-glutamine when glucose levels drop too low. It is the most abundant amino acid, and it helps stabilize mental functioning and promotes a sense being alert and calm. Several studies show that concentrations of glutamine in the body are diminished during times of stress. Symptoms of deficiency include depression, moodiness, irritability, increased food cravings, lack of focus and concentration, anxiety, and insomnia.

Dosage: 500–3000 mg daily.

Chromium picolinate

Chromium picolinate is a mineral used to help the regulation of insulin as well as blood sugar and fat metabolism. It has been shown to effectively moderate sugar and carbohydrate cravings.

Dosage: 200–400 mcg daily.

DL-phenylalanine

DL-phenylalanine is classified as an essential amino acid. It can be converted to tyrosine, which in turn is converted to neurotransmitters dopamine, norepinephrine, epinephrine, and thyroid hormones. Phenylalanine is found in three forms: L-phenylalanine, the natural form found in proteins in foods; D-phenylalanine, a mirror image of L-phenylalanine that is made in a laboratory; and DL-phenylalanine, a combination of the two forms. The different forms of phenylalanine have been proposed to treat depression and mood disorders, food cravings, lack of energy, memory problems, and appetite regulation.

Dosage: 100–250 mg daily.

N-acetyl-L-cysteine

N-acetylcysteine (NAC) stimulates glutathione synthesis, promotes liver detoxification, and is a powerful antioxidant that supports the system during stress, infections, toxic assault, and inflammatory conditions. A growing body of research has found that NAC can reduce cravings for highly addictive substances like cocaine, heroin, and cigarettes. It also reduces compulsive behaviour problems such as gambling, overeating, or impulsive-compulsive eating disorders such as bulimia.

Dosage: 600–1200 mg twice daily to curb cravings.

Cravings most often accompany mood disorders such as depression and bipolar disorder, so it is important to review the nutritional support recommendations mentioned earlier. In addition, these disorders are often exacerbated by stress, so if you feel stress is a factor in your life, you would benefit from stress support.

 LOOK for a product such as...

Stress Less, that contains the adaptogenic herbs ashwagandha, rhodiola, and *Panax ginseng.* (Refer to Chapter 2 for more information on stress, stressors, and stress support.) In addition, remember the importance of supporting the three brains with the **Daily Brain,** packet. The three brains are involved in most of the common mental health disorders.

PGX®

PGX, as previously mentioned, helps regulate blood sugar, a factor involved in many different mental health disorders. People who have blood sugar imbalances often experience abnormal sugar or carbohydrate cravings.

Dosage: 750–1500 mg before each meal.

ADHD in Adults

About 4% of adults experience some or all ADHD symptoms. It affects men and women almost equally. The various possible causes of ADHD and other learning disorders in adults are the same as in children and adolescents. A recent study done at the Mayo Clinic showed that ADHD persists into adulthood, as 30% of people who were diagnosed with it had it as a child. They also had a greater risk for other mental health issues, like anxiety, depression, antisocial personality disorder, and substance abuse.

ADHD can be harder to diagnose in adults due to the following:

- Other mental health disorders can cause problems with concentration and cause restlessness and impulsivity. More than three-quarters of adults living with ADHD have another mental illness, including depression, bipolar disorder, social anxiety disorder, substance use disorders, and personality disorders.

- Clinicians may have less training to recognize ADHD in adults.

- Adults are more able to develop coping strategies that hide symptoms. For example, an adult who feels very restless can choose a busy, fast-paced job or change jobs often.

Supplement Support for Adults with ADHD

Stress and stress hormones have been found to be a major factor in people with ADD/ADHD. (Refer to Chapter 2 for information on the effects of stress.) If you feel stress is a factor in your life and could be contributing to lack of mental focus, confusion, or anxiety-like symptoms, it would be wise to consider adding a formula that contains adaptogens to help regulate stress hormones.

 LOOK for a product such as...

Stress Less, which contains ashwagandha, rhodiola, *Panax ginseng,* green tea extract, and choline.

Supplements that are helpful in children with learning disorders and ADHD are also beneficial for adults. Refer to Chapter 6 for treatment suggestions for supplement support for ADHD. In addition, refer to the dietary guidelines outlined in Chapter 5 as a foundation for healing brain disorders.

Sleep Disorders and the Three Brains

According to Statistics Canada, one in seven Canadians have insomnia, the inability to fall asleep, stay asleep, or experience restorative sleep. The World Association of Sleep Medicine states that sleep problems, including insomnia, sleep apnea, restless legs syndrome, and sleep deprivation in general, affect up to 45% of the world's population. It claims that 60% of Canadian adults feel tired most of the time and get, on average, 6.9 hours of sleep a night, despite the fact that experts recommend eight hours. Canadian research indicates that 30% of adults get fewer than six hours of sleep a night. Chronic sleep deprivation can contribute to obesity, diabetes, high blood pressure, heart attack, stroke, depression, decreased immunity, and inflammatory and other medical conditions.

Not only are adults struggling to cope with an epidemic of sleep disorders, but doctors are also observing alarming rates of sleepiness and sleeplessness in children. "As many as 40% of Canadian children aren't getting enough sleep, which is not only impairing their ability to function properly, it's hurting their ability to learn", said Dr. Reut Gruber of Montreal's Douglas Mental Health University Institute. Health care practitioners suggest teenagers need about nine hours of sleep a night, while children in elementary school should be getting 10–12 hours a night.

Insomnia

Insomnia is one of the most common sleep disorders seen in medical practice, and treatment of this condition is challenging and often unsatisfactory for the patient. Severe insomnia is defined as the difficulty initiating or maintaining sleep at least three times a week for one month or longer, with the problem being bad enough to cause fatigue or impaired functioning during the day. Insomnia has always been and still is under-recognized. It is an under-treated problem since about 60% of the people suffering from insomnia never talk to their health care practitioners about their sleeping difficulties.

Common Causes of Insomnia

There are many possible causes of insomnia.

- **Psychological conditions:** Sleep disturbance is a common feature of emotional disorders. For example, 90% of depressed people have insomnia. However, insomnia is also a major risk factor for depression. It is often unclear which condition triggers the other.

- **Gut-Brain inflammation:** Anxiety and depression are common causes of insomnia and new research shows a direct link between gut microbiota and mental health disorders such as anxiety and depression.

- **Alcohol:** An estimated 10–15% of chronic insomnia cases result from substance abuse, especially alcohol, cocaine, and sedatives. For most people, one or two drinks a day pose no problem and may even help initiate sleep.

- **Medical conditions:** Several conditions contribute to or cause insomnia, including chronic pain (e.g., arthritis, back pain), cardiovascular disease, respiratory diseases, gastrointestinal disorders, hormone conditions, and some neurological conditions. In one survey, 22% of adults reported that health conditions, pain, or discomfort impaired their sleep.

- **Medications:** Several medications cause insomnia. If your insomnia seems to be associated with when you started taking a medication, talk to your health care practitioner.

- **Nightly leg problems:** Leg disorders that occur at night, such as restless leg syndrome or leg cramps, are very common and are an important cause of insomnia.

- **Shift work:** Shift work throws off the body's circadian rhythm and may lead to chronic insomnia.

- **Blood sugar imbalances:** Blood sugar imbalances are also a common – though less recognized – cause of insomnia. Adrenal compromised individuals commonly have blood sugar problems ranging from hypoglycemia (low blood sugar) to hyperglycemia (high blood sugar). Low blood sugar at night results in restless sleep, bizarre dreams, and poor sleep quality for the entire night. One of the mechanisms the body will call on to liberate more glucose is to increase cortisol and adrenaline, which will convert stored fats and carbohydrates into sugars for immediate use. The increase in blood sugar sends more sugar to the brain, causing a restless, light sleep during the night. Coffee and alcohol exacerbate the problem, while eating a small protein meal before bed can help regulate blood sugar levels.

- **Menopause:** Another type of insomnia very commonly seen is sleep disturbances as a result of the menopausal transition. Some women wake up due to hot flashes at night, sometimes followed by episodes of chilling. For others, insomnia is independent of hot flashes. Once hormones are regulated, sleeping problems will improve for most women.

- **Sleep apnea:** It is important to rule out sleep apnea in anyone suffering with insomnia. This breathing disorder results in brief interruptions of breathing during sleep. Some individuals will experience snoring in-between these pauses, while others will describe a choking sensation. People with sleep apnea experience periods of anoxia (oxygen deprivation of the brain) with each episode. The most common treatment of sleep apnea is the continuous positive airway pressure (CPAP) machine. Testing is often done through a referral to a sleep clinic through your health care practitioner.

> Elevated cortisol due to stress and HPA dysregulation is a main cause of chronic insomnia. Insomnia worsens HPA dysregulation and increases cortisol, resulting in a vicious cycle that is difficult to control.

The Stress-Sleep Connection

Stressful life events are closely associated with the onset of chronic insomnia. Stress plays a leading role in the hypothalamic-pituitary-adrenal (HPA) axis dysregulation and the associated increase in cortisol and norepinephrine (NE) play a primary role in some sleep disorders. In other cases, the HPA axis dysfunction is actually the result of a sleep disorder, as seen in obstructive sleep apnea.

The effect of sleep disorders on cortisol levels

The daily rhythm of cortisol secretion is influenced by the circadian clock. Sleep, particularly deep sleep, has an inhibitory effect on cortisol secretion, while sleep disruptions are accompanied by cortisol stimulation. Consistent research shows an elevation in cortisol levels following even partial sleep loss. After only one night of sleep restricted to four hours, plasma cortisol levels were 37% higher the following day. Even if sleep deprivation is modest, it causes a profound disruption in the daily cortisol rhythm, resulting in activation of the HPA axis, associated with sleep disturbances.

In the not too distant past, it was thought that sleep loss had no ill-health effects, apart from daytime sleepiness. More recent research has overturned this belief and has shown that sleep loss (less than seven hours per night) may have wide-ranging effects on the cardiovascular, endocrine, immune, and nervous systems. Some of the common conditions potentially caused by sleep problems include obesity in adults and children, chronic pain symptoms, diabetes and glucose intolerance, cardiovascular disease, hypertension, cognitive impairments, anxiety, and depression.

The effect of cortisol levels on sleep disorders

The main stress hormone cortisol has a natural rhythm – normally peaking between 6 am and 8 am. Then, between 8 am and 11 am, cortisol levels begin to drop and gradually decline throughout the day, reaching the lowest point about 2 am. The cyclical rise and fall of cortisol levels govern our level of wakefulness throughout the day and night. Cortisol is excitatory; it arouses us and wakes us up which is great in the morning. But, when cortisol levels get stuck at higher levels as a result of prolonged stress, it is bad news for a good night's sleep.

Stress is associated with the activation of the HPA axis, causing increased cortisol, and resulting in arousal and sleeplessness. Studies have shown that cortisol levels are significantly higher in insomniacs compared to normal sleepers. So we know that stress-induced dysfunction of the HPA axis and elevated cortisol play a significant role in sleep disorders, but in other cases, the HPA axis dysfunction may be a result of a sleep disorder. Which came first? Or does it matter? Either way, it is a vicious cycle for people suffering from chronic insomnia.

Later in this chapter we will offer suggestions for how to stop this cycle.

Other Brain Chemicals and Hormones Affecting Chronic Insomnia

Abnormal levels of certain brain chemicals have been observed in some people with chronic insomnia.

- **The cortisol-melatonin relationship:** In adults, melatonin onset typically occurs during low cortisol secretion, which under normal circumstances would be at night. However, as mentioned previously, chronic stress causes an increase in cortisol in the evening, resulting in decreased secretion of melatonin, one of the body's sleep hormones. Also, with aging, the production of melatonin declines and is shifted to later hours, while the production of cortisol increases and its peak occurs earlier in the night. Perhaps this is where the mistaken belief that older people need less sleep comes from. It is not that the elderly need less sleep, it is simply that aging can cause dysregulation in cortisol and melatonin secretions.

- **Cortisol and gamma-aminobutyric acid (GABA):** GABA is synthesized in the brain and cortisol has a dual action on the GABA receptors. Lower levels of cortisol enhance concentrations of GABA, while higher levels of cortisol inhibit GABA. GABA is the most important inhibitory neurotransmitter in the brain, acting like a "brake" during times of runaway stress. Decreased GABA function in the brain is associated with several neurological disorders, including anxiety, depression, insomnia, and epilepsy.

- **Thyroid disorders:** It is common knowledge that hyperthyroidism (excess of thyroid hormone) is strongly associated with insomnia. The excess thyroid hormone causes anxiety, fast heart rate, and hyper arousal of the nervous system. One study showed that after only six days of four-hour sleep time, thyroid-stimulating hormone (TSH) levels were strikingly decreased, and overall mean TSH levels were reduced by more than 30%. Therefore, if you have long-term chronic insomnia and have never been tested for thyroid problems, you might want to consider it. (Refer to Chapter 5 for more information on thyroid disorders and thyroid testing.)

The Mental-Emotional-Physical Cycle

In addition to the sleep deprivation/HPA/cortisol cycle, many people experience emotional responses to chronic insomnia. The resulting cycle becomes even more self-perpetuating. The emotional response added to the physical cause (i.e., dysregulation of the HPA axis, chronic pain) is called psychophysiological insomnia. This occurs as follows:

- An episode of transient insomnia disrupts the person's circadian rhythm.

- The person begins to associate the bed not with rest and relaxation, but with a struggle to sleep, causing added stress. From here a deeper pattern of sleep failure emerges.

> Unless you have experienced cycles of chronic insomnia, it is very difficult to understand just how utterly devastating it is!

- Over time, this event repeats, and bedtime becomes a source of anxiety. The person is stressed about the inability to sleep, the consequences of sleep loss, the lack of mental control, and the overall debilitating effects. All attempts to sleep fail.

- Eventually excessive worry about sleep loss becomes persistent and provides an automatic nightly trigger for anxiety and arousal, and insomnia becomes self-perpetuating, lasting indefinitely.

PERSONAL STORY

When I was 48 years old, my life changed when I started suffering from chronic insomnia. Up until then I had the energy to meet all the increasing demands in my life. You could say I was like the "ever ready battery that never quits". I had a very demanding naturopathic clinic, was writing books, and was travelling for public presentations almost every weekend. I also had my family responsibilities as a single parent with three sons.

When the insomnia started, I was absolutely exhausted on every level, and I had to push hard just to barely function throughout the day. By evening, my adrenal glands had finally responded, but at the wrong time of the day, with an overproduction of stress hormones. I was tired, and all I wanted was sleep. My body was exhausted and "running on empty", but my brain was wired and sleep was impossible. I was the classic case of "tired but wired". To be honest, many times I wondered if I could carry on, as the physical, mental, and emotional effects were absolutely devastating. Keeping people awake is truly a form of torture – it breaks them.

My insomnia was a result of years of cumulative demands and stress: raising three sons as a single mom, medical school, lack of money, incapacitating back pain, and the demands of my career, on top of seven years spent in a very stressful personal relationship. Further complicating matters were the extra demands on my adrenals during the hormonal changes at menopause; my adrenals just decided they had had enough. I had been diagnosed with adrenal fatigue in my early thirties, and for the most part had managed to keep them supported to meet the demands, but not this time.

For the first year of my insomnia cycle I refused to take anything other than naturopathic remedies, but it just wasn't enough. I would sit on the floor in my bedroom and rock and cry all night. I would finally fall asleep around 5 am and I had to be up by 7 am. The stress of the insomnia put even more stress on my adrenal glands, and things went from bad to worse. Finally I realized I needed to do whatever it took to break this vicious cycle.

It took a long time for me to find an effective prescription medication that didn't make me feel "hung over". Most often the side effects were worse than not sleeping. However, once my sleep started to improve there was less stress on my nervous system, and over time, I was able to rely on natural supplements to help me with sleep. Even now, 20 years later, I sometimes have to take my prescription medications for a few days during times of increased stress or travel, when the naturopathic remedies are not quite enough. However, now I know that it won't be forever, and if I don't stop the vicious stress-sleep cycle early, it will become even more difficult to break. My advice is to do whatever you need to do to break the cycle.

Support Recommendations for Insomnia

An effective way to manage sleep problems due to cortisol dysregulation is to ensure the adrenal glands are supported by proper nutrition. In fact, adrenal regulation is necessary in order to stop the vicious cycle of stress and insomnia. Insomniacs and those who feel "tired but wired" should take most supplements – including adrenal support – in the morning. Look for a product that contains adaptogenic herbs such as ashwagandha, ginseng, and rhodiola, as well as choline and an antioxidant like green tea extract. (Refer to Chapter 2 for more information on stress and stress support.)

People who have anxiety or feel wired during the day should use a calming support such as GABA and or L-theanine to prevent anxiety often associated with insomnia. Take this in the early afternoon and evening to keep the nervous system calm and prevent overstimulation. While the adrenal glands are getting the help they need, most people with insomnia will need additional support specific for sleep needs.

Stress is a very real factor for many people with insomnia. It is important to add stress reduction support to help prevent the overproduction of stress hormones that can keep you wired even though you are exhausted from lack of sleep.

 LOOK for a product such as...

Stress Less, which helps prevent overproduction of stress hormones. (Refer to Chapter 2 for more information on stress.)

Supplement Support for Insomnia

Passion flower *(Passiflora incarnate)*

Passion flower has been used traditionally for anxiety disorders, general nervousness, attention-deficit hyperactivity disorder (ADHD), and insomnia. Several controlled studies have demonstrated enhanced sleep benefits for adults with insomnia.

Dosage: 500–1000 mg daily of a 4:1 extract.

California poppy *(Eschscholzia californica)*

California poppy is used for insomnia, mood disorders, nervous agitation, and to promote relaxation. It is also effective for pain relief, specifically nerve pain.

Dosage: 1000–2000 mg daily of a 4:1 extract at night.

Hawthorn *(Crataegus)*

Hawthorne has been used traditionally as a cardiovascular tonic. New research indicates that hawthorn has antioxidant properties and is effective in treating stress-related disorders such as nervousness and anxiety that are often the underlying cause of insomnia. This herb is usually used in combination with other herbs in the treatment of insomnia.

Dosage: 125–250 mg daily of a 4:1 extract.

Linden flowers *(Tillia cordata)*

Traditionally, linden flowers have been used to soothe nerves and to treat conditions associated with stress, including anxiety and insomnia.

Dosage: 100–200 mg daily of a 5:1 extract.

Skullcap *(Scutellaria lateriflora)*

Skullcap has been used for centuries as relaxant and as a therapy for anxiety, nervous tension, and insomnia. Studies show that American skullcap has significant antioxidant effects, and may help protect against disorders such as Alzheimer's disease, anxiety, and depression.

Dosage: 2000–4000 mg daily.

Valerian *(Valeriana officinalis)*

Valerian has been proven beneficial for sleep disorders, especially those associated with stress and anxiety. In a double-blind comparison study involving patients 18–73 years of age diagnosed with insomnia, two groups were treated with either 600 mg daily of valerian extract or 10 mg daily of oxazepam (benzodiazepine). Sleep quality after six weeks in those taking valerian extract was at least as effective as the oxazepam treatment. Both treatments markedly increased sleep quality compared with baseline. Adverse events occurred in

28.4% receiving valerian extract and 36.0% taking oxazepam, and were all rated mild to moderate. No serious adverse drug reactions were reported in either group. Most patients assessed their respective treatment as very good (82.8% in the valerian group, 73.4% in the oxazepam group).

Dosage: 400–700 mg daily of a solid root extract one hour before bed.

GABA

GABA is the most important inhibitory neurotransmitter in the brain. It acts like a brake in times of increased stress, eliciting a sense of calm. Low levels of GABA have been linked to anxiety, depression, and insomnia. GABA increases the production of alpha brainwaves characterized by being relaxed, as well as greater mental focus and alertness. It also reduces beta waves associated with nervousness and hyperactivity. In addition, it has been shown to produce relaxation by reducing stress markers such as heart rate, cortisol levels, and pupil diameter.

Dosage: 100–200 mg 2–3 times daily. As a general guideline, it is recommended to take no more than 3000 mg within a 24-hour period.

Melatonin

Melatonin helps maintain the body's circadian rhythm, an internal 24-hour clock that plays a critical role in when we fall asleep and when we wake up. The body produces more melatonin when it is dark and less when it is light. Being exposed to bright lights too late in the evening can disrupt melatonin production. Older people typically exhibit poor sleep due to reduced melatonin levels. A double-blind placebo-controlled study examined the effects of melatonin in doses ranging from 1–3 mg in subjects over 50 years of age. Both doses improved sleep.

Dosage: start with 1–2 mg at bedtime and if necessary increase up to 5 mg.

Magnesium glycinate

Magnesium has been found to be effective for treating depression and anxiety, insomnia, short-term memory loss, irritability, and agitation. People suffering from headaches also benefitted from magnesium supplementation.

Dosage: 200–400 mg daily.

5-hydroxytryptophan

5-Hydroxytryptophan (5-HTP) may prove to be better than melatonin at treating insomnia. Several clinical studies have shown 5-HTP to produce good results in promoting and maintaining sleep in normal subjects as well as those experiencing insomnia. In many cases, insomnia has been associated with tryptophan deficiency in the tissues of the brain. Tryptophan is the precursor to 5-HTP, which is then converted into serotonin and then into melatonin.

Dosage: 100–300 mg daily.

 LOOK for a product for insomnia such as...

Restful Sleep, containing important herbs such as passion flower, California poppy, skullcap, and linden flower.

For more stubborn cases of insomnia, additional support may be required during the day:

- Stress is a very real factor for many people with insomnia. It is important to add stress reduction support to help prevent the overproduction of stress hormones that can keep you wired even though you are exhausted from lack of sleep. A product such as Stress Less can help keep you calm, yet alert during the day. (Refer to Chapter 2 for more information on stress support.)

- If you are still feeling anxious or stressed, consider taking GABA or L-theanine mid-to-late afternoon to provide additional calm to the nervous system. (See information in the anxiety section earlier in this chapter.)

Medications for Insomnia to Help Break the Vicious Cycle

There is a time and a place for every medical philosophy. Sometimes pharmaceuticals are not only necessary, but life-saving. For those who suffer from debilitating insomnia and who find that natural products are not helping, prescription medicine may be necessary to break the cycle at different periods of time. This will depend on the individual. Once the sleep cycle begins to improve, it is time to try natural sleep remedies. Begin by taking less of the prescription medication along with a natural product.

If prescription medications prove to be necessary, it is important to support the adrenal glands and address any accompanying anxiety with the supplements mentioned above. The underlying causes need to be addressed despite the medications providing relief from symptoms. Improvements in the adrenals can take months for some, depending on the level of ongoing stress.

Tips for Dealing with Insomnia

Most people who have chronic insomnia have tried all of the "sleep tips" and will get frustrated and tired of hearing the most basic and logical of suggestions. For those who suffer from occasional insomnia, some of the following tips may be helpful:

- Cut out stimulants by avoiding caffeinated beverages (coffee, chocolate, tea, soft drinks) past noon.
- Do not exercise in the evening as this can cause cortisol levels to increase in people with adrenal fatigue.
- Do not eat a large meal late in the evening (after 7 pm). Try to avoid snacking after dinner.
- Keep your fluid intake high during the day and less at night to avoid having to get up in the night to urinate.
- Take a hot bath before bed (unless it aggravates hot flashes if you are a menopausal woman). Add calming essential oils such as lavender and chamomile.
- Take time for meditation, contemplation, or prayer before you retire.

In this stressful world, it is often hard to find time for yourself. When there is a window, the "brain chatter" often takes over with reminders of all the things on the "to do" list. Everyone has something that they find both physically and mentally calming, the inner quiet time where the brain is quiet and the body is more relaxed. Whether it is a walk in nature, yoga, meditation, being mesmerized by watching water, climbing a mountain, or listening to relaxing music, just do it! If you have a full schedule, make an appointment with yourself that you can't cancel. After all, you are the most important item on the "to do" list.

Memory Disorders

In 2011, 15% of Canadians 65 or older were living with cognitive impairment, including dementia. This year alone, more than 100,000 Canadians will be diagnosed with dementia – that is one person every five minutes. It is estimated that 5.3 million people in the US have Alzheimer's disease and by 2020 that number is expected to balloon to 7.1 million, representing a 40% percent increase in less than a decade.

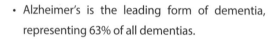

- Alzheimer's is the leading form of dementia, representing 63% of all dementias.

- Vascular dementia is second, representing 20% of all dementias.

- Women represent 72% of Alzheimer's cases and 47% of vascular dementia.

- Less than 10% people have early-onset dementia.

Alzheimer's is the most common type of dementia. Dementia is an umbrella term describing a variety of diseases and conditions that develop when nerve cells in the brain (called neurons) die or no longer function normally. The death or malfunction of neurons causes changes in memory, behaviour, and the ability to think clearly.

Types of Dementia

Vascular Dementia

Vascular dementia is a general term describing problems with reasoning, planning, judgment, memory, and other thought processes. It is caused by brain damage from impaired blood flow from the brain.

Vascular dementia can occur after a stroke blocks an artery in the brain, but strokes don't always cause vascular dementia. Whether a stroke affects thinking and reasoning depends on its severity and where it occurs in the brain. Vascular dementia can also be caused by other conditions or treatments that damage blood vessels and reduce circulation, depriving your brain of vital oxygen and nutrients.

Alzheimer's Disease

There are three types of Alzheimer's.

- **Early-onset Alzheimer's:** This rare form of Alzheimer's affects people before the age of 65. Less than 10% of the people with Alzheimer's have this form of the disease. Early-onset Alzheimer's appears to be linked with a genetic defect, whereas late-onset Alzheimer's is not.

- **Late-onset Alzheimer's:** This is the most common form of Alzheimer's, accounting for about 90% of all cases. It usually occurs after age 65. The neuronal loss and atrophy occurs principally in the frontal cortex and temporal lobe, which houses the hippocampus. Several studies have demonstrated that pro-inflammatory substances accompany the deposition of plaque called beta-amyloid proteins, which is the signature of Alzheimer's.

- **Familial Alzheimer's:** This form of Alzheimer's is entirely inherited. It is very rare and accounts for less than 1% of all cases. Familial Alzheimer's can occur as early as the late thirties or early forties.

Protein tangles and plaques in Alzheimer's

Tau is a protein found inside brain cells. Its role is to provide a structure to help the cells clear any accumulation of unwanted and toxic proteins. Fewer plaques accumulate outside the brain cells when tau is functioning. Plaques are an accumulation of sticky proteins called beta-amyloid. The death of brain cells begins when tau fails to function properly. When tau is abnormal, these proteins, which include beta-amyloid, accumulate inside the neurons. Essentially, the proteins begin to exert toxic effects inside the cell, so the cells do their best to spit out the proteins into the extracellular space. The beta-amyloid protein fragments are sticky, so they begin to clump together into plaque.

The protein that can't be spit out and remains inside the neurons is what destroys them – not the plaques building up on the outside of the cells. The cell cannot remove the garbage, and this garbage includes beta-amyloid as well as tau. Meanwhile, the beta-amyloid released from the dead neuron sticks to the plaque and adds to its bulk. Researchers have found that without the interaction of toxic beta-amyloids with tau, the Alzheimer's cascade cannot begin. People who suffer from Alzheimer's show plaques and tangles (twisted strands of tau) inside the brain.

Dementia with Lewy Bodies

Lewy bodies are clumps of protein similar to beta-amyloid plaques, but which contain a different protein. These form in the cortex of the brain, not the hippo-campus as in Alzheimer's.

Early Symptoms of Dementia

People developing dementia may exhibit the following symptoms:

- Memory loss affecting day-to-day function, such as forgetting phone numbers (even your own), appointments, a colleague's name, etc.

- Difficulty performing familiar tasks such as preparing a meal, or becoming so distracted that you forget to turn off the stove

- Problems with language such as finding the right words – even simple words – and making substitutions that don't make sense

- Disorientation of time and place, such as becoming lost in a familiar area and not knowing how to get home, or not knowing what month it is

- Poor judgment, such as wearing cold-weather clothing on a warm day, or not recognizing a condition that needs medical attention

- Problems with abstract thinking, such as balancing a chequebook or being able to pay bills

- Misplacing things on a regular basis, or putting things in inappropriate places, such as the phone in the freezer

- Changes in mood, behaviour, or personality (e.g., going from tears to anger for no apparent reason, feelings of confusion or suspicion, being withdrawn and apathetic, feeling extremely fearful over nothing)

People with Alzheimer's seem to have more dramatic personality changes and anger outbursts than people with vascular dementia.

Possible Causes of Dementia

Although there is a connection between family history and genetics for some people, many other factors have been linked to the development of dementia, including Alzheimer's.

Metabolism

Multiple clinical observations have demonstrated that dementia in general, and Alzheimer's in particular, are associated with type 2 diabetes and obesity. Moreover, type 2 diabetes is considered an independent risk factor for dementia, with the prevalence of dementia in diabetic populations double that of healthy patient populations. Researchers have shown that individuals with Alzheimer's have a lower concentration of insulin in their cerebrospinal fluid and a higher concentration in their blood than controls, both of which indicate impaired insulin metabolism in the brain. Based on the results of these studies, Alzheimer's could be considered as a metabolic disease, with progressive impairment of the brain's capacity to use glucose and respond to insulin.

Insulin treatment improves memory and attention span and lowers the concentrations of the amyloid precursor protein. This protein has been implicated in the development of Alzheimer's, which is now being referred to as type 3 diabetes.

- Metabolic disturbances have been implicated in neurodegenerative disorders, including Alzheimer's, Huntington's, and Parkinson's diseases. Multiple clinical observations have demonstrated that dementia in general, and Alzheimer's in particular, are associated with type 2 diabetes and obesity. Moreover, type 2 diabetes is considered an independent risk factor for dementia. The prevalence of dementia in diabetic populations is double that of healthy patient populations.

- Researchers have shown that individuals with Alzheimer's have a higher concentration of insulin in their which indicates impaired insulin metabolism in the brain. Based on these results, Alzheimer's could be considered a metabolic disease, with progressive impairment of the brain's capacity to use glucose and respond to insulin. Some experts are now referring to Alzheimer's as type 3 diabetes.

- Metabolic syndrome is an important factor in the development of mild cognitive impairment, vascular dementia, and Alzheimer's. Stress hormones, inflammation, and oxidative stress contribute to an insulin-resistant brain state, causing decreased glucose metabolism and the formation of beta-amyloid and tau proteins, both signatures of Alzheimer's.

Inflammation

- Inflammation is the cornerstone of Alzheimer's, Parkinson's disease, multiple sclerosis, and other autoimmune disorders. Researchers have found that systemic inflammation leads to the production of pro-inflammatory cytokines in the hippocampus region of the brain. This region is involved in memory and learning.

- A UK study published in the *Journal of Biological Psychiatry* in 2010 suggested inflammation in the brain may accelerate the progress of dementia. The research team found that just one episode of systemic inflammation (whole body inflammation) could be sufficient to trigger a more rapid decline in neurological function. The researchers found that systemic inflammation leads to the production of a pro-inflammatory cytokine by the brain's immune cells in the hippocampus region of the brain. This region is involved in memory and learning.

- Alzheimer's and generalized cognitive decline are marked by age-related brain changes, such as disturbed immune function, and increased oxidative stress which contribute to inflammation. These factors are influenced by diet and the gut microbiota. In addition, brain-derived neurotrophic factor, which protects and encourages the survival of healthy brain cells and whose production is influenced by gut bacteria, is shown to be decreased in people with Alzheimer's.

Head and Heart Brain Connection in Dementias

Growing evidence suggests that the health of the brain is closely linked to the overall health of the heart and blood vessels. A healthy heart helps ensure that enough blood is pumped through these blood vessels to the brain, and healthy blood vessels help ensure that the brain is supplied with the oxygen- and nutrient-rich blood it needs to function normally.

Vascular dementia is associated with decreased blood flow to the brain. Cerebral blood flow is automatically regulated, allowing maintenance of a constant blood supply over a wide range of blood pressure. This regulatory mechanism shifts in the elderly, which can allow for rapid changes in blood pressure. Hypertension (increase in blood pressure) has been recognized as a risk factor for vascular dementia, but more recent studies show that lesions in the brain and cognitive decline can also be caused by a rapid fall in blood pressure.

New evidence suggests a strong link between dementias and heart disease, and there also seem to be many similarities between the two diseases. Research has shown that the same risk factors that result in cardiovascular disease, such as high blood pressure, cholesterol, and obesity, put people at higher risk for dementias, including Alzheimer's. These risk factors lead to atherosclerosis, a process where deposits of cholesterol and other substances (plaques) build up in the arteries and narrow the blood vessels. Researchers have found that this process not only occurs in the cardiovascular system, but also in the brain. Atherosclerosis can lead to heart attack causing blood clots, and may also lead to dementias by reducing the flow of blood that nourishes the brain. You may recall that inflammation is at the root of atherosclerosis. (Refer to Chapter 3 for more information on inflammation.)

Free Radical Damage

Excessive free radical damage is now thought to be a major player not only in brain aging and traumatic brain injury, but also in degenerative conditions like Alzheimer's and in mild cognitive impairment. As cognitive function begins to decline, markers for free radical damage correlate directly with the degree of mental impairment. (Refer to Chapter 6 for more information on how to protect the brain from free radical damage.)

Traumatic Brain Injury

Traumatic brain injury (TBI) is the disruption of normal brain function caused by a blow or jolt to the head or penetration of the skull by a foreign object. Moderate TBI is associated with twice the risk of developing Alzheimer's and other dementias compared with no head injuries, and severe TBI is associated with 4.5 times the risk.

Gluten Intolerance and the Gut Brain Connection

Gluten, which is in most carbohydrates such as breads, pastas, and cereals, might cause inflammation in the brain. Grains also cause an increase in blood sugar, and even slight elevations in blood sugar can increase the risk of developing dementia.

Dr. David Permutter, well-known neurologist and author of *Grain Brain*, says: "The biggest issue by far is that carbohydrates are absolutely at the cornerstone of all of our major degenerative conditions". He adds, "That includes things like Alzheimer's, heart disease, and even cancers. What we know is that even mild elevations in blood sugar are strongly related to developing Alzheimer's. Even mild elevations in blood sugar compromise brain structure and lead to shrinkage of the brain. That's what our most well-respected, peer-reviewed journals are telling us". In addition to gluten, other food intolerances or allergies can affect brain function and memory. (Refer to Chapter 4 for more information on gluten and allergies and the brain.)

Stress

Stress hormones appear to rapidly exacerbate the formation of brain lesions and the progression of dementias, including Alzheimer's. Management of both physical and psychological stress is crucial in the prevention and treatment of this devastating disease. The hippocampus is the primary area of degeneration in Alzheimer's. Stress hormones are toxic to the nerve cells, and stress-mediated glucocorticoids, whether too high or too low, reduce the size and plasticity of the hippocampus.

Researchers showed that when animals were injected for just seven days with stress hormones, the levels of the different proteins in the brain increased by 60%. These proteins, called beta-amyloids, form plaques or tangles in the brain, another signature of Alzheimer's. However, so far the drugs that remove these proteins have not succeeded in arresting the steady decline of thinking and memory. (Refer to Chapter 2 for more information on stress and the three brains.)

Gut Microbiota Imbalances

In addition to the stress factor, neurodegenerative diseases such as Alzheimer's and generalized cognitive decline are marked by age-related brain changes, disturbed immune function, and increased oxidative stress, which are influenced by diet and abnormal gut microbiota. The imbalance in the microbiota interferes with the production of a brain-derived neurotrophic factor (BDNF) that protects and encourages survival of healthy brain cells. This BDNF is decreased in people with Alzheimer's. We know that depression and dementia are closely connected, so it is notable that the unhealthy dietary patterns that negatively influence the gut microbiota are also risk factors for depression.

Pesticides

New evidence published in March 2014 in *JAMA Neurology* suggests that pesticides and Alzheimer's could be intricately linked. The research showed that 74 out of the 86 Alzheimer's patients studied had blood levels of DDE (a toxic chemical compound) almost four times higher than those of the 79 people in the control group who did not have Alzheimer's. Patients with a version of ApoE gene (ApoE4), which greatly increases the risk of developing Alzheimer's, along with high blood levels of DDE, exhibited even more severe cognitive impairment than the patients without the risk gene. Epidemiological studies also show evidence that DDT/DDE affect pathways associated with the development of beta-amyloid plaques, a hallmark of Alzheimer's. Other contaminants such as heavy metals (aluminum) and chemicals in the water, soil, or air are also thought to be involved in dementias.

Telomeres

Each time a cell replicates, a small piece of the DNA is removed from each chromosome. As these telomeres shorten, it affects genetic expression, resulting in degenerative conditions such as Alzheimer's. Curcumin has been shown to prevent the shortening of telomeres.

Elevated Homocysteine Levels

Elevated homocysteine levels occur in approximately one third of people over 61 years of age. This risk factor is estimated to account for 22% of the instances of Alzheimer's.

The rate of brain atrophy is associated with elevated levels of homocysteine, an essential amino acid that regulates phospholipid metabolism. Elevated homocysteine inhibits this process and, as a result, less omega-3 fatty acids are incorporated into phosphatidylcholine (PC). Decreased omega-3 content of PC has been linked to Alzheimer's disease.

B vitamins, particularly B6, B12, and folic acid, reduce levels of homocysteine and one study showed a nine-fold reduction in brain shrinkage and a substantial reduction in rate of memory loss with the addition of these vitamins. In subjects with above average omega-3 levels, B vitamins reduced brain atrophy rates by 40% and improved Hopkins Verbal Learning Test (HVLT) scores. The HVLT assesses verbal learning and memory.

Patrick Holford is an expert in nutrition who specializes in mental health and memory disorders. He stresses the importance of nutrition and supplementation for optimal brain function. His foundation, Food for the Brain (www.foodforthebrain.org), promotes awareness of the connection between learning, behaviour, mental health, and nutrition.

Thyroid Disorders

A clinically detectable over- or underactive thyroid has long been recognized as a cause of cognitive (thinking, learning, and memory) impairment. Research shows that older women who have high or low levels of TSH have more than twice the risk of developing Alzheimer's than those with more moderate thyroid hormone levels.

Thyroid hormone function is intricately linked to the central nervous system: adults with hypothyroidism are more prone to depression, whereas those with hyperthyroidism are subject to confusion. Recent studies have also related thyroid dysfunction to an increased risk for irreversible dementia. Today, thyroid dysfunction is significantly underdiagnosed in clinical practice. As a result of recent research, it has been suggested that the current TSH levels (typically 0.5–5.0 mIU/L) should be adjusted to a narrower range of 0.3–3.04 mIU/L. (Refer to Chapter 4 for more information on thyroid disorders and the three brains.)

Undiagnosed low thyroid epidemic affects a possible 70% of the population, causing serious health problems. A study by Dr. E. Chester Ridgeway, the University of Colorado's chief endocrinologist, stated that an estimated 13 million Americans may have undiagnosed thyroid problems, up from previous estimates. He says that even mild thyroid problems might cause serious consequences. Pregnant women with underactive thyroid are in jeopardy of having children with lower IQs. Research shows that low thyroid levels can raise cholesterol levels, thus raising the threat of a heart attack. In his April 10, 2000 news release, Dr. Ridgeway said that "people don't realize what a big problem this is and how important it is to get the word out".

Other Possible Causes

Apart from neurodegenerative disease like dementias or neurological diseases, other medical conditions may also lead to an impairment of memory. Diabetes, insomnia, obesity, thyroid disorders, obstructive sleep apnea, and hormonal changes are examples of non-dementia conditions that can cause memory impairment.

Brain atrophy has been associated with diabetes, and hypoglycemia due to insulin therapy may also lead to memory impairments. TBI survivors often suffer from long-term memory impairment as a consequence, and mood disorders such as depression are often accompanied by cognitive deficits not related to dementias. However, depressive patients also suffer from structural abnormalities, such as reduced hippocampus volume, which may be reversible during remission.

Many people, particularly the aging, are taking a mix of pharmaceuticals that can contribute to memory disorders. A broad range of medications may cause or increase memory impairment, including benzodiazepines, antipsychotics, opioids, anticonvulsants, glucocorticoids (steroids), some antidepressants, analgesics (pain medications)and anticholinergics (statins), pointing to the importance of a detailed drug history in patients who complain of memory deficits.

Ways to Preserve Cognition

Mediterranean Diet

New research suggests that adherence to the Mediterranean diet may prevent brain atrophy and thereby preserve cognition in the elderly. Participants who adhered more to a Mediterranean diet had larger brain volumes both in grey matter and white matter, associated with the higher intake of fish and lower intake of meat. Potential mechanisms include anti-inflammatory and/or antioxidative effects, as well as potential slowing of the accumulation of beta-amyloid or tau proteins. David Knopman, MD, professor of neurology at the Mayo Clinic College of Medicine in Rochester, Minnesota, said the finding that diet may influence brain volume is novel and adds a "dimension of biology" to the hypothesis that diet and brain health are linked. (Refer to Chapter 5 for more information on the Mediterranean diet.)

Preventing Conditions Associated with Alzheimer's

For many people, it may be possible to prevent Alzheimer's by doing what you can to prevent the conditions associated with it. For example, insulin resistance, diabetes, hypertension, and heart disease all increase the risks. In most cases, these conditions are preventable and/or treatable. In addition, if dementia is a concern due to family history, chronic stress, toxic exposure, or medical history, review the supplements that can help prevent inflammation and provide nutritional support for the brain.

Tests That Could Help Save Your Head and Heart Brains

Lab tests for inflammation or cardiovascular risk factors should be considered to determine possible risk factors for dementia. Elevated C-reactive protein and homocysteine levels appear to be independent risk factors for cognitive decline. Testing for the ApoE4 genotype, or the Alzheimer's gene, should be considered for those who have a family history of Alzheimer's. Monitoring blood sugar and blood pressure are important, as well as testing thyroid, salivary cortisol, and B12 levels. (Refer to Chapter 4 for information on these lab tests.)

The "smell test" maintains that when you lose the ability to sense certain smells, like lemon, leather, natural gas, or strawberry, you are at a much greater risk for Alzheimer's. This loss of ability means the neurons in the olfactory (smell) centres are dying. Smell identification tests may be available from your health care practitioner.

These measures will not guarantee that you will not get dementia or forms of memory loss, but they will certainly lower the risk. According to one study from the Veterans Affairs Hospital in San Francisco, preventing the diseases associated with Alzheimer's decreases the incidence by 50%.

Supplement Support for Memory Disorders

Huperzine A *(Huperzia serrata)*

A randomized, double-blinded, placebo-controlled study was done with Huperzine A in vascular dementia patients. After 12 weeks of treatment, the test assessment scores significantly improved in the Huperzine A group, whereas the placebo group did not show any improvement. The researchers concluded that Huperzine A can significantly improve the cognitive function in patients with mild-to-moderate vascular dementia.

Dosage: 10–20 mg daily of an extract standardized to 1% Huperzine A.

Alpha-lipoic acid

Oxidative stress plays a crucial role in age-related neurodegenerative disorders. One study with mice examined alpha-lipoic acid (ALA) and N-acetyl-L-cysteine (NAC) in animals with cognitive deficits. Administration of either LA or NAC improved cognition, indicating the therapeutic role of antioxidants in supporting cognitive function.

Dosage: 300–600 mg daily.

N-acetyl-L-cysteine

N-acetyl-L-cysteine (NAC) has been shown to be effective in the treatment of Alzheimer's and some other brain disorders. This effect may be directly associated with the inflammatory pathway and/or working through oxidative processes associated with inflammation. In addition to the effects on oxidative balance, alterations in cysteine levels have also been shown to modulate neurotransmitter pathways, including glutamate.

Dosage: 400–800 mg daily.

Phosphatidylserine

With the increasing aging population and cognitive and memory problems in general, the work of Dr. Thomas Crook, internationally recognized memory expert, is important to consider. Dr. Crook states that phosphatidylserine (PS) can slow, halt, or reverse the decline of memory and mental function due to aging. In a double-blind trial, Crook and his team found that administering 300 mg of PS daily could restore up to 12 years' worth of lost mental function. Studies using PET scanning to investigate brain glucose use in Alzheimer's patients noted increased glucose use in PS-supplemented patients. PS may also protect cells from damage produced by free radicals. Elderly patients showed significant improvements in behavioural alterations (loss of motivation, initiative, interest in the environment, and socialization), memory, and learning in the PS group compared to placebo. At least a dozen other studies note similar significant improvements in learning, memory, concentration, and recall.

Dosage: 300 mg daily.

> "Some people object quite strongly to the idea that age-associated memory impairment is a condition that requires treatment. They argue that it is a normal sign of aging. However, if a middle-aged man can't read the newspaper anymore, we don't tell him to go away, we provide reading glasses. If someone has thin bones, we give them drugs to protect them against fractures even though bone-thinning is normal in old age. So why are we more hesitant to treat 'normal' age-related memory loss now that we have the tools to do so successfully? I have been involved in researching a number of different memory treatments and nothing else comes close to PS." – Thomas H. Crook III, PhD.

Acetyl-L-carnitine

Studies show that acetyl-L-carnitine increases synaptic connections in the brain and consequently improves learning capacity. It is able to travel through the blood-brain barrier, where it then helps protect brain cells from free radical damage and is a precursor for the synthesis of the neurotransmitter acetylcholine.

Dosage: 500–1000 mg 1–3 times daily.

Vinpocetine (periwinkle)

Vinpocetine increases blood circulation and glucose metabolism, and reduces brain impairment after ischemic stroke. Other studies have shown improved cognitive effects even in patients who have had multiple cerebral blockages, leading researchers to conclude that vinpocetine is effective in the treatment of vascular dementia.

Dosage: 5–10 mg 3 times daily.

Ginkgo biloba

This powerful antioxidant is often associated with increased cerebral blood flow and enhanced memory. Catechins, procyanidins, and flavonoids are important components of standardized extracts of ginkgo. These active components were found to be potent inhibitors of beta-amyloid aggregation, and are able to destabilize the exiting plaques.

Dosage: 150–250 mg daily of a standardized extract.

Note: Contraindicated in people taking blood thinners such as Coumadin.

In addition to Daily Brain for three-brain support, people with memory problems will require additional nutritional supplementation.

LOOK for a product such as...

Memory Boost, that combines important memory support supplements such as N-acetyl-L-cysteine, alpha-lipoic acid, ginkgo, vinpocetine, phosphatidylserine (PS), phosphatidylcholine (PC), phosphatidylethanolamine (PE), and huperzia.)

In addition to taking a supplement providing the ingredients mentioned above, it is important to prevent and/or treat the inflammation that is the cause of many memory disorders.

Curcumin *(Curcuma longa)*

Curcumin is a potent anti-inflammatory that can prevent and help treat the inflammatory cause of Alzheimer's. It also has antioxidant, lipophilic, and metal chelation effects. It plays a significant role in the treatment of dementias, including Alzheimer's, as well as other brain disorders such as depression, and symptoms related to traumatic brain injuries. (Refer to Chapter 3 for more information on inflammation and the brain.) Another protective effect of curcumin may be its effect on telomerase expression. In a study published in the *Journal of Alzheimer's Disease*, curcumin demonstrated the ability to enter the brain, bind, and destroy the beta-amyloid plaques present in Alzheimer's, with reduced toxicity.

Dosage: 300 mg 2–3 times daily of an extract standardized to 33% curcuminoids.

Boswellia *(Boswellia serrata)*

Boswellia, also known as Indian frankincense, has been used as an anti-inflammatory agent for centuries. Many studies have shown that it is as effective as non-steroidal anti-inflammatory drugs, which are the most common treatment for inflammatory conditions.

Dosage: 300–500 mg 2–3 times daily of an extract standardized to 30–40% boswellic acids.

Ashwagandha *(Withania somnifera)*

This powerful adaptogen has been used in Ayurvedic medicine (one of the world's oldest holistic healing systems, developed in India) for over 3,000 years. Clinical trials and animal research support the use of ashwagandha for anxiety, cognitive and neurological disorders, brain injuries, inflammation, and neurodegenerative diseases such as dementia and Alzheimer's. Ashwagandha has been shown to regenerate brain cells, and preliminary research has found that it also inhibits the formation of beta-amyloid plaques. It does not alter brain chemistry, but rather boosts a protein in the liver that clears amyloid from the brain.

Dosage: 125–250 mg 1–2 times daily of an extract standardized to 8% withanolides.

Bacopa *(Bacopa monnieri)*

This herb supports the nervous system and the adrenals, the stress adaptive organs. It has been used historically to strengthen the immune response and increase the ability to cope with physical and mental stress. It provides antioxidant protection for memory centres and reduces the effects of stress on the brain. Bacopa improves cognitive performance, anxiety, and depression, and reduces amyloid deposits in the brain.

Dosage: 200 mg 1–2 times daily.

Note: This dosage applies only if the total bacoside content (active compound) is 55% of the extract. To achieve the ideal 10–20% bacoside content, 750–1500 mg of the leaf or powder is required.

 LOOK for a product such as...

Brain Defence, to help with inflammation and cognition that combines bacopa, ashwagandha, curcumin, boswellia, and chamomile to support cognition, and to prevent and treat inflammation.

Omega-3 fatty acids

Studies show that omega-3 fatty acids protect the brain from damages related to oxidative stress (free radical damage). A number of studies have shown that reduced intake of omega-3 fatty acids is associated with increased risk of age-related cognitive decline or dementia, including Alzheimer's. Scientists believe the omega-3 fatty acid docosahexaenoic acid (DHA) is protective against Alzheimer's and dementia. It is thought that DHA might enhance cognitive abilities by facilitating synaptic plasticity and/or enhancing synaptic membrane fluidity; it might also act through its effects on metabolism, as DHA stimulates glucose use and mitochondrial function, reducing oxidative stress.

Dosage: 1000–3000 mg daily.

Multivitamins

A multivitamin is very important to supply the necessary cofactors for optimal brain function. This is particularly important in the elderly where diet and food choices do not always provide the necessary minerals and vitamins.

Dosage: depends on the type of product. Follow the manufacturer's instructions.

B12 and folic acid

B12 promotes normal memory, concentration, and verbal function. B12 and folic acid help maintain normal homocysteine levels for healthy cognitive function. Older people may not produce enough stomach acid to process the vitamin B12. People with vitamin B12 deficiency are more likely to score lower on cognitive tests, as well as have a smaller total brain volume, which suggests a lack of the vitamin may lead to brain shrinkage. Studies have shown that those with the lowest B12 levels had a six-fold greater rate of brain volume loss compared with those who had the highest levels. Interestingly, none of the participants were actually deficient in vitamin B12 – they just had low levels within a normal range. This goes to show that normal is not necessarily the same as optimal. One of the researchers stated, "Our results suggest that rather than maintaining one's B12 at a level that is just above the cut-off for deficiency, it might be prudent to aim to keep it higher up than normal range". Symptoms of vitamin B12 deficiency include numbness and tingling of the extremities, especially the legs; difficulty walking; concentration problems; memory loss; disorientation; and dementia that may or may not be accompanied by mood changes.

Dosage: B12: 1000–2000 mcg daily; folic acid: 1–2 mg daily.

Vitamin E

Vitamin E has been shown to reduce the problems of memory loss and learning in the aging population. A study in the January 1, 2014 issue of the *Journal of the American Medical Association* showed that 2000 IU of vitamin E significantly delayed clinical progression in patients with mild-to-moderate Alzheimer's.

Dosage: 400–800 IU daily.

Alpha-glycerylphosphorylcholine

Alpha-glycerylphosphorylcholine (GPC) has been shown to be effective in reducing the loss of neuro-connecting fibres and brain cells. GPC is an extremely bioavailable source of choline, which is a building block of acetylcholine, which decreases with age. GPC has been linked with helping memory loss due to low acetylcholine levels. Studies have shown significant improvement in memory and overall function in patients with dementias.

Dosage: 1200 mg daily.

Pyrroloquinoline quinone

Pyrroloquinoline quinone (PQQ) is a vitamin-like compound found in plant foods that has shown a wide range of benefits. It is an extremely powerful antioxidant that provides defence against decay as well as growth of new mitochondria, the cell's energy producers. Mitochondrial dysfunction is a key biomarker of aging and is definitively linked to the development of virtually all diseases of aging, from Alzheimer's, Parkinson's, and type 2 diabetes, to heart failure. PQQ protects brain cells against oxidative stress and neurotoxicity induced by other powerful toxins, and protects nerve cells from the damaging effects of the beta-amyloid protein linked with Alzheimer's. Overall, it protects against memory and cognition decline.

Dosage: 20 mg daily.

LOOK for a product such as...

Brilliant Mind, that contains omega-3 fatty acids, phosphatidylserine, phosphatidylcholine, Alpha-glycerophosphorylcholine (Alpha-GPC), and green tea for added support for the aging brain.

Water

Water is essential for optimal brain function. Water prevents dehydration, increases blood circulation, aids in the removal of toxins, and keeps the brain from overheating – all factors that contribute to cognitive decline and even nerve cell damage. Dehydration can lead to fatigue, dizziness, poor concentration, and reduced cognitive abilities. Even mild levels of dehydration affect mental performance.

Exercise

Studies have shown significant increases in brain volume in both grey and white matter regions of the brain in older adults who participated in aerobic fitness training, but not for those who participated in stretching and toning (non-aerobic). No significant changes in either grey or white matter volume were detected for younger participants. This study strongly suggests a positive role for aerobic fitness in maintaining and enhancing brain health and cognitive functioning in older adults.

New studies are providing even more evidence that regular aerobic exercise not only prevents problems with memory that come with aging, but can actually help turn back the clock on brain aging. Researchers at the Mayo Clinic found that moderate exercise in mid-life is associated with a 39% reduced chance of developing cognitive impairment. Furthermore, moderate exercise in late life is associated with a 32% reduction in the odds of mental decline. Moderate exercise includes exercise such as brisk walking, aerobics, yoga, strength training, and swimming. Try incorporating one or more of these activities into your regular routine four times per week for 20–30 minutes. A growing body of literature supports the benefits of a physically active lifestyle in general, but also on the brain. Exercise decreases inflammation and increases healthy gut bacteria – both factors that have positive benefits on brain health.

> I read a Dutch study that said, "Backward locomotion appears to be a very powerful trigger to mobilize cognitive resources". Because my grandmother, my mother, and my aunt all had varying degrees of dementia, I want to do all I can to prevent it from happening to me. One day, as I was walking up a hill backward, a truck stopped and the driver asked what I was doing. I said, "I am trying to prevent Alzheimer's disease". The driver then said, "Sorry to tell you but you are too late lady!" Well, whether walking backwards will prevent Alzheimer's or not, it is a great way to use muscles you don't know you have, and it's good for a few laughs, too!

Brain Games – Use It or Lose It

Several different brain training or brain games promote neuroplasticity and help with optimal performance. Brain fitness requires variety and curiosity. Most of us like familiarity, but when anything you do becomes rote or second nature, then you need to make a change. Try something new! Take a new route to work, go to a different grocery store, or try a new type of exercise.

Brain fitness games are also a good way to challenge your brain. Sudoku, crossword puzzles, Internet or electronic games, and card games like bridge can all exercise your brain. These games rely on logic, word skills, math, and more. Try to find 15–20 minutes a day to exercise your brain.

Anti-Inflammatory Foods

Inflammation is a primary cause of memory loss and dementia. In addition to supplementation with Theracurmin or boswellia, a range of foods provide extra protection from inflammation:

- **Omega-3 fats** – Found in fatty fish like wild Alaskan salmon, krill, mackerel, sardines, and black cod, as well as in fish oil and krill oil, these fats help fight inflammation and are particularly important for brain health. Research published in 2012 the *Scandinavian Journal of Gastroenterology* confirmed that dietary supplementation with krill oil effectively reduced inflammation and oxidative stress.

- **Leafy greens** – Dark leafy greens such as kale, spinach, collard greens, and Swiss chard contain powerful antioxidants, flavonoids, carotenoids, and vitamin C, all of which help protect against cellular damage. Ideally, opt for organic locally grown veggies that are in season, and consider eating some of them raw, particularly in the summer months. Juicing is an excellent way to get more greens into your diet.

- **Blueberries** – Blueberries are a good source of antioxidants compared to other fruit and vegetables. They are also lower in sugar than many other fruit.

- **Tea** – Matcha tea is the most nutrient-rich green tea. It comes in the form of a stone-ground unfermented powder and has up to 17 times the antioxidants of wild blueberries.

- **Fermented vegetables and traditionally cultured foods** – These foods help optimize your gut flora, which is important for a well-functioning immune system. They also help ward off chronic inflammation. In fact, the majority of inflammatory diseases start in your gut as the result of an imbalanced microbiome. Fermented foods such as kefir, kimchee, miso, tempeh, pickles, sauerkraut, and other fermented vegetables, will help recolonize the gut with beneficial bacteria. Fermented foods can also help your body rid itself of harmful toxins such as heavy metals and pesticides that promote inflammation.

- **Shiitake mushrooms** – These mushrooms contain strong compounds with the natural ability to discourage inflammation and inhibit oxidative stress.

- **Garlic and onions** – Garlic has been shown to work similarly to non-steroidal anti-inflammatory pain medications (like ibuprofen), shutting off the pathways that lead to inflammation. Onions contain similar anti-inflammatory chemicals, including the phytonutrient quercetin and the compound allicin, which break down to produce free radical-fighting sulfenic acid.

- **Nuts and seeds** – Nuts and seeds help fight inflammation, particularly almonds, which are rich in fibre, calcium, and vitamin E, and walnuts, which have high amounts of alpha-linolenic acid, a type of omega-3 fat. All nuts contain high levels of antioxidants, which can help your body fight off and repair the damage caused by inflammation.

- **Olive oil** – The Mediterranean diet's many health benefits may be largely due to its liberal use of olive oil, especially the extra-virgin kind. The compound oleocanthal, which gives olive oil its taste, has been shown to have a similar effect to nonsteroidal anti-inflammatory painkillers in the body.

- **Berries** – All fruit can help fight inflammation because they are low in fat and calories and high in antioxidants. Berries in particular have been shown to have anti-inflammatory properties, possibly because of anthocyanins (antioxidants), the powerful chemicals that give them their rich colour. Animal studies have shown that red raspberry extract helps arthritis, and blueberries can help protect against intestinal inflammation and ulcerative colitis. Women who eat more strawberries have lower levels of C-reactive protein.

- **Tart cherries (sour cherries)** – Oregon Health & Science University researchers suggest that tart cherries have the highest anti-inflammatory content of any food. Studies have found that tart cherry juice can reduce the inflammation in blood vessels by up to 50%, and it has been shown to reduce people's use of anti-inflammatory pain medication. Experts recommend eating 355 g (1.5 cups) of tart cherries, or drinking 235 mL (about 1 cup) of tart cherry juice daily to see similar benefits. Sweet cherries don't seem to have the same effects.

- **Avocado** – This creamy fruit is considered the most perfect food in the world. It is loaded with fibre and vitamins, and is an excellent source of healthy fats. Dr. Perlmutter, a neurologist and author of the book Grain, considers the avocado part of his "anti-Alzheimer's trio", along with coconut oil and grass-fed beef.

Memory loss and cognitive impairment are not part of the normal aging process. While cognitive decline may be caused by brain lesions associated with Alzheimer's, these changes are not inevitable and it is entirely possible to prevent damage from occurring in the first place by reducing brain busters such as stress as much as possible, and by following the dietary and supplement guidelines.

References

SECTION 1
Chapter 1

Anderson P. Does Parkinson's begin in the gut? *Medscape Medical News*. 2012 June. Available from http://www.medscape.com/viewarticle/765675.

Armour, JA. Potential clinical relevance of the "little brain" on the mammalian heart. *Exp Physiol*. 2008; 93(2):165-76.

Bercik, P, Denou E, Collins J, et al. The intestinal microbiota affect central levels of brain-derived neurotropic factor and behavior in mice. *Gastroenterology*. 2011; 141(2):599-609.

Bercik P, Verdu EF, Foster JA, et al. Chronic gastrointestinal inflammation induces anxiety-like behavior and alters central nervous system biochemistry in mice. *Gastroenterology*. 2010; 139(6):2102-12.

Bravo JA, Forsythe P, Chew MV, et al. Ingestion of Lactobacillus strain regulates emotional behavior and central GABA receptor expression in a mouse via the vagus nerve. *Proc Natl Acad Sci USA*. 2011; 108(38):16050-5.

Cartin, M, Genest J. The heart as an endocrine gland. *Sci Am*. 1986; 254(2):62-7.

Corcoran CD, Thomas P, Phillips J, et al. Vagus nerve stimulation in chronic treatment-resistant depression. Preliminary findings of an open-label study. *Brit J Psychiat*. 2006; 189(3):282-3.

Dash SR. The microbiome and brain health: what's the connection? *Medscape*. 2015 Mar. Available from http://www.medscape.com/viewarticle/841748.

Del Arco A, Mora F. Neurotransmitters and prefrontal cortex-limbic system interactions: implications for plasticity and psychiatric disorders. *J Neural Transm*. 2009; 16(8):941-52.

Foster JA, McVey Neufeld KA. Gut-brain axis: how the microbiome influences anxiety and depression. *Trends Neurosci*. 2013; 36(5):305-12.

Hadhazy A. Think twice: how the gut's "second brain" influences mood and well being. *Sci Am*. Feb 12, 2010; 95.

Johnson, EJ. A possible role for lutein and zeaxanthin in cognitive function in the elderly. *Am J Clin Nutr*. 2012 Nov; 96(5):1161S-5S.

Madsen K. Probiotics and the immune response. *J Clin Gastroenterol*. 2006; 40:232-4.

Mastone R. The neuroscience of the gut. *Sci Am,* April 19. 2011; 23.

McCraty R, Atkinson M, Bradley RT. Electrophysiological Evidence of intuition: part 1. The surprising role of heart. *J Altern Complem Med*. 2004; 10(1):133-43.

Messaoudi M, Lalonde R, Violle N, et al. Assessment of psychotropic-like properties of a probiotic formulation (*Lactobacillus helveticus* R0052 and *Bifidobacterium longum* R0175) in rats and human subjects. *Br J Nutr*. 2011; 105(5):755-64.

Mulle JG, Shapr, WG, Cubells JF, et al. The gut microbiome: a new frontier in autism research. *Curr Psychiatry Rep*. 2013; 15(2):337.

Prindle A, Liu J, Asally M, et al. Ion channels enable electrical communication in bacterial communities. *Nature;* Nov 5 2015; 527:59-63.

Roberfroid MB. Prebiotics and probiotics: Are they functional foods? *Am J Clin Nutr*. 2000; 71:1682S–7S. [PubMed]

Samuels MA. Contemporary reviews in cardiovascular medicine. The brain-heart connection. *Circulation*. 2007; 116:77-84.

Wu JY, Prentice H. Role of taurine in the central nervous system. *J Biomed Sci*. 2010; 17(Suppl 1):S1.

Xu Y, Lin D, Li S, et al. Curcumin reverses impaired cognition and neuronal plasticity induced by chronic stress. *Neuropharmacology*. 2009; 57(4):463-71.

Chapter 2

Auddy B, Hazra J, Mitra A, et al. A standardized *Withania somnifera* extract significantly reduces stress-related parameters in chronically stressed humans: a double-blind, randomized, placebo-controlled study. *JANA*. 2008; 11:50-6.

Buydens-Branchey L, Branchey, M, Hibbeln JR, et al. Associations between increases in plasma n-3 polyunsaturated fatty acids following supplementation and decreases in anger and anxiety in substance abusers. *Prog Neuropsychopharmacol Biol Psychiatry*. 2008; 32(2):568-75.

Coleman CI, Hebert JH, Reddy P. The effects of *Panax ginseng* on quality of life. *J Clin Pharm Ther*. 2003; 28(1):5-15.

Darbinyan V, Kteyan, A, Panossian, A, et al. *Rhodiola rosea* in stress induced fatigue – a double blind cross-over study of a standardized extract SHR-5 with a repeated low-dose regimen on the mental performance of healthy physicians during night duty. *Phytomedicine*. 2000; Oct; 7(5):365-71.

Eby GA, Eby KL. Magnesium for treatment-resistant depression: a review and hypothesis. *Med Hypotheses*. 2010; 74(4):649-60.

Institute of Food Technologists (IFT). Eight nutrients to protect the aging brain. *ScienceDaily*. 15 April 2015. Available from http://www.sciencedaily.com/releases/2015/04/150415203340.htm.

Jensen K, Schauch M. *Stress and the disease connection: a complete guide*. Hillsburgh ON: ActNatural Corporation; 2015.

Kalman DS, Feldman S, Feldman R, et al. Effect of a proprietary magnolia and phellodendron extract on stress levels in healthy women: a pilot, double-blind, placebo-controlled clinical trial. *Nutr J*. 2008; 7:11.

Kaufer D. Stress and glucocorticoids promote oligodendrogenesis in the adult hippocampus. *Mol Psychiatry*. 2014; 19:1275-83.

REFERENCES

Kiecolt-Glaser JK, Belury MA, Andridge R, et al. Omega-3 supplementation lowers inflammation and anxiety in medical students: a randomized controlled trial. *Brain Behav Immun.* 2011; 25(8):1725-34.

Mishra LC, Singh BB, Dagenais S. Scientific basis for the therapeutic use of *Withania somnifera* (ashwagandha): a review. *Altern Med Rev.* 2000; 5(4):334-46.

Murray MT. *Stress, anxiety and insomnia: what the drug companies won't tell you and your doctor doesn't know.* Coquitlam BC: Mind Publishing; 2012.

Nakagawa K, Kuriyama K. Effect of taurine on alteration in adrenal functions induced by stress. *Jpn J Pharmacol.* 1975; 25(6):737-46.

Qu WM, Yue XF, Sun Y, et al. Honokiol promotes non-rapid eye movement sleep via the benzodiazepine site of the GABA(A) receptor in mice. *Br J Pharmacol.* 2012; 167(3):587-98.

Rai D, Bhatia G, Sen T, et al. Anti-stress effects of *Ginkgo biloba* and *Panax ginseng*: a comparative study. *J Pharmacol Sci.* 2003; 93(4):458-64.

Schmidt K, Cowen PJ, Harmer CJ, et al. Prebiotic intake reduces the waking cortisol response and alters emotional bias in healthy volunteers. *Psychopharmacology.* 2015; 232(10):1793-801.

Shevtsov VA, Zholus BI, Shervarly VI, et al. A randomized trial of two different doses of a SHR-5 *Rhodiola rosea* extract versus placebo and control of capacity for mental work. *Phytomedicine.* 2003; 10(2-3):95-105.

Singal A, Kaur S, Tirkey N, et al. Green tea extract and catechin ameliorate chronic fatigue-induced oxidative stress in mice. *J Med Food.* 2005; 8(1):47-52.

Talbott SM, Talbott JA, Pugh M. Effect of *Magnolia officinalis* and *Phellodendron amurense* (Relora®) on cortisol and psychological mood state in moderately stressed subjects. *J Int Soc Sports Nutr.* 2013; 10(1):37.

SECTION 2

Chapter 3

Ammon HP. Boswellic acids in chronic inflammatory diseases. *Planta Med.* 2006; 72(2):1100-16.

Bell S, Grochoski GT, Clarke AJ. Health implications of milk containing beta-casein with the A2 genetic variant. *Crit Rev Food Sci Nutr.* 2006; 46(1):93-100.

Benros ME, Waltoft BL, Nordentoft M, et al. Autoimmune diseases and severe infections as risk factors for mood disorders: a nationwide study. *JAMA Psychiatry.* 2013; 70(8):812-20.

Berchtold NC, Chinn G, Chou M, et al. Exercise primes a molecular memory for brain-derived neurotrophic factor protein induction in the rat hippocampus. *Neuroscience.* 2005; 133(3):853-61.

Bravo JA, Forsythe P, Chew MV, et al. Ingestion of *Lactobacillus* strain regulates emotional behavior and central GABA receptor expression in a mouse via the vagus nerve. *Proc Natl Acad Sci.* 2011; 108(38):16050-5.

Cohen S, Janicki-Deverts D, Doyle WJ, et al. Chronic stress, glucocorticoid receptor resistance, inflammation, and disease risk. *Proc Natl Acad Sci.* 2012; 109(16):5995-9.

Colantuoni C, Rada P, McCarthy J, et al. Evidence that intermittent excessive sugar intake causes endogenous opioid dependence. *Obes Res.* 2000; 10(6):478-88.

Cryan, JF, O'Mahony SM. The microbiome-gut-brain axis: from bowel to behavior. *Neurogastroenterol Motil.* 2011; 23(3):187-92.

Cuaz-Pérolin C, Billiet L, Baugé E, et al. Anti-inflammatory and antiatherogenic effects of the NF-kappaB inhibitor acetyl-11-keto-beta-boswellic acid in LPS-challenged ApoE-/- mice. *Arterioscler Thromb Vasc Biol.* 2008; 28(2):272-7.

Dantzer, R, O'Connor JC, Freund GG, et al. From inflammation to sickness and depression: when the immune system subjugates the brain. *Nat Rev Neurosci.* 2008; 9(1):46-56.

Dobos N, Korf J, Luiten PGM, et al. Neuroinflammation in Alzheimer's disease and major depression. *Biol Psychiatry.* 2010; 67(6):503-4.

Fasano A. Physiological, pathological, and therapeutic implications of zonulin-mediated intestinal barrier modulation: living life on the edge of the wall. *Am J Pathol.* 2008; 173(5):1243-52.

Fasano, A. Zonulin and its regulation of intestinal barrier function: the biological door to inflammation, autoimmunity, and cancer. *Physiol Rev.* 2011; 91(1):151-75.

Gayathri B, Manjula N, Vinaykumar KS, et al. Pure compound from *Boswellia serrata* extract exhibits anti-inflammatory property in human PBMCs and mouse macrophages through inhibition of TNF-alpha, IL-1beta, NO and MAP kinases. *Int Immunopharmacol.* 2007; 7(4):473-82.

Hadjivassiliou, M. Gluten sensitivity as a neurological illness. *J Neurol Neurosurg Psychiatry.* 2002; 72(5):560-3.

Jackson JR, Eaton WW, Cascella NG, et al. Neurologic and psychiatric manifestations of celiac disease and gluten sensitivity. *Psychiatr Q.* 2012; 83(1):91-102.

Jyonouchi H, Geng L, Ruby A, et al. Evaluation of an association between gastrointestinal symptoms and cytokine production against common dietary proteins in children with autism spectrum disorders. *J Pediatr.* 2005; 146(5):605-10.

Kang JX, Weylandt KH. Modulation of inflammatory cytokines by omega-3 fatty acids. *Subcell Biochem.* 2008; 49:133-43.

Kirste S, Treier M, Wehrle SJ, et al. *Boswellia serrata* acts on cerebral edema in patients irradiated for brain tumors: a prospective, randomized, placebo-controlled, double-blind pilot trial. *Cancer.* 2011; 117(16):3788-95.

Kohler O, Benros ME, Nordentoft M, et al. Effect of anti-inflammatory treatment on depression, depressive symptoms, and adverse effects: a systematic review and meta-analysis of randomized clinical trials. *JAMA Psychiatry.* 2014; 71(12):1381-91.

Kumamoto CA. Inflammation and gastrointestinal *Candida* colonization. *Curr Opin Microbiol*. 2011; 14(4):386-91.

Lopresti AL, Hood SD, Drummond PD. Multiple antidepressant potential modes of action of curcumin: a review of its anti-inflammatory, monoaminergic, antioxidant, immune-modulating and neuroprotective effects. *J Psychopharmacol*. 2012; 26(12):1512-24.

Maroon JC, Bost JW. Omega-3 fatty acids (fish oil) as an anti-inflammatory: an alternative to nonsteroidal anti-inflammatory drugs for discogenic pain. *Surg Neurol*. 2006; 64(4):326-31.

Mysels DJ, Sullivan MA. The relationship between opioid and sugar intake: review of evidence and clinical applications. *J Opioid Manag*. 2010; 6(6):445-52.

Okusaga O, Yolken RH, Langenberg P, et al. Elevated gliadin antibody levels in individuals with schizophrenia. *World J Biol Psychiatry*. 2015; 14(7):509-15.

O'Mahony SM, Clarke G, Borre YE, et al. Serotonin, tryptophan metabolism and the brain-gut-microbiome axis. *Behav Brain Res*. 2015; 277:32-48.

Setiawan E, Wilson AA, Mizrahi R, et al. Role of translocator protein density, a marker of neuroinflammation, in the brain during major depressive episodes. *JAMA Psychiatry*. 2015; 72(3):268-75.

Shehzad A, Rehman G, Lee YS. Curcumin in inflammatory diseases. *Biofactors*. 2013; 39(1):69-77.

Simopoulos AP. Omega-3 fatty acids in inflammation and autoimmune diseases. *J Am Coll Nutr*. 2002; 21(6):495-505.

Slavich GM, Irwin MR. From stress to inflammation and major depressive disorder: a social signal transduction theory of depression. *Psychol Bull*. 2014; 140(3):774-815.

Spangler R, Wittkowski KM, Goddard NL, et al. Opiate-like effects of sugar on gene expression in reward areas of the rat brain. *Brain Res Mol Brain Res*. 2004; 124(2):134-42.

Tillisch K, Labus J, Kilpatrick L, et al. Consumption of fermented milk product with probiotic modulates brain activity. *Gastroenterology*. 2013; 144(7):1394-401.

Chapter 4

Caricilli A, Saad M. The Role of Gut Microbiota on Insulin Resistance. *Nutrients*. 2013 Mar; 5(3): 829-851.

Beyreuther K, Biesalski HK, Fernstrom JD, et al. Consensus meeting on monosodium glutamate. *Eur J Clin Nutr*. 2007; 61(3):304:13.

Crane, K. *A wellness guide for the digital age*. Global Wellbeing Books; 2014.

Environmental working group. EWG's guide to safer cell phone use: executive summary. 27 Aug 2013. Available from www.ewg.org/research/cellphoneradiation/executive summary.

Frisardi V, Solfrizzi V, Capurso C, et al. Is Insulin resistant brain state a central feature of the metabolic-cognitive syndrome? *Alzheimers Dis*. 2010:21(1):57-63.

Grandjean P, Landrigan PJ. Neurobehavioural effects of developmental toxicity. *Lancet*. 2014; 13(3):330-8.

Kleinriddersa A, Caia W, Cappelluccib L, et al. Insulin resistance in brain alters dopamine turnover and causes behavioral disorders. *Proceedings of the National Academy of Sciences (PNAS)*. 2015; 112(11):3463-68.

Lauritano EC, Bilotta AL, Gabrielli M,et al. Link between hypothyroidism and small intestinal bacterial overgrowth. *J Clin Endocrinol Metab*. 2014; 18(3):307-9.

Maillard P, Seshadri S. Effects of systolic blood pressure on white-matter integrity in young adults in the Framingham Heart Study: a cross-sectional study. *Lancet*. 2012; 11(12):1039-47.

Mittag J, Lyons DJ, Sällström J, et al. Thyroid hormone is required for hypothalamic neurons regulating cardiovascular functions. *J Clin Invest*. 2013; 123(1):509-16.

Mori, K. Does the gut microbiota trigger Hashimoto's thyroiditis? *Discovery Medicine*. November 27, 2012. Available from http://www.discoverymedicine.com/Kouki-Mori/2012/11/27/does-the-gut-microbiota-trigger-hashimotos-thyroiditis/.

Patil, AD. Link between hypothyroidism and small intestinal bacterial overgrowth. *Indian J Endocrinol Metab*. 2014 May-Jun; 18(3):307-9.

Pelton R, LaValle JB, Hawkins EB. *Drug-induced nutrient depletion handbook*. 2nd Ed. Ohio: Lexi-Comp; 2001.

Sharma M, Kupferman JC, Brosgol Y, et al. The effects of hypertension on the paediatric brain: a justifiable concern. *Lancet Neurol*. 2010; 9(9):933-40.

Spinasanta S. *Untreated hypothyroidism, thyroid hormone, and cardiac effects*. The Endocrine Society's 97th Annual Meeting, 6 Mar 2015. Available from http://www.endocrineweb.com/professional/meetings/thyroid-hormone-effects-cardiac-function.

Wium-Andersen MK, Orsted DD, Nielsen SF, et al. Elevated C-reactive protein levels, psychological distress, and depression in 73,131 individuals. *JAMA Psychiatry*. 2013; 70(2):176-54.

Wu A, Ying Z, Gomez-Pinilla F. Dietary omega-3 fatty acids normalize BDNF levels, reduce oxidative damage, and counteract learning disability after traumatic brain injury in rats. *J Neurotrauma*. 2004; 21(10):1457-67.

SECTION 3

Chapter 5

Bavarsad Shahripour R, Harrigan MR, Alexandrov AV. N-acetylcysteine (NAC) in neurological disorders: mechanisms of action and therapeutic opportunities. *Brain Behav*. 2014; 4(2):108-22.

Benton D. Dehydration influences mood and cognition: a plausible hypothesis? *Nutrients*. 2011; 3(5):555-73.

Brand-Miller JC, Atkinson FS, Gahler RJ, et al. Effects of PGX®, a novel functional fibre, on acute and delayed postprandial glycaemia. *Eur J Clin Nutr*. 2010; 64(12):1488-93.

Cenacchi T, Bertoldin T, Farina C, et al. Cognitive decline in the elderly: a double-blind, placebo-controlled multicenter study on efficacy of phosphatidylserine administration. *Aging Clin Exp Res*. 1993; 5(2):123-33.

REFERENCES

Chang CY, Ke DS, Chen JY. Essential fatty acids and human brain. *Acta Neurol Taiwan*. 2009; 18(4):231-41.

Chung SY, Moriyama T, Euzu E, et al. Administration of phosphatidylcholine increases brain acetylcholine concentration and improves memory in mice with dementia. *J Nutr*. 1995; 125(6):1484-9.

Colcombe SJ, Erickson K. Aerobic exercise training increases brain volume in aging humans. *J Gerontol A Biol Sci Med Sci*. 2006; 61(11):1166-70.

Crook TH, Petrie W, Well C, et al. Effects of phosphatidylserine in Alzheimer's disease. *Psychopharmacol Bull*.1992; 28(1):61-6.

Crook TH, Tinklenberg J, Yesavage J, et al. Effects of phosphatidylserine in age-associated memory impairment. *Neurology*. 1991; 41(5):644-9.

Davison K, Berry NM, Misan GM, et al. Dose-related effects of flavanol-rich cocoa on blood pressure. *J Hum Hypertens*. 2010; 24(9):568-76.

De Nicolo S, Tarani L, Ceccanti M, et al. Effects of olive polyphenols administration on nerve growth factor and brain-derived neurotrophic factor in the mouse brain. *Nutrition*. 2013; 29(4):681-7.

De Vriese SR, Christophe AB, Maes M. Lowered serum n-3 polyunsaturated fatty acid (PUFA) levels predict the occurrence of postpartum depression: further evidence that lowered n-PUFAs are related to major depression. *Life Sci*. 2003; 73(25):3181-7.

Desideri G, Kwik-Uribe C, Grassi D, et al. Benefits in cognitive function, blood pressure, and insulin resistance through cocoa flavanol consumption in elderly subjects with mild cognitive impairment: the Cocoa, Cognition, and Aging (CoCoA) study. *Hypertension*. 2012; 60(3):794-801.

Eby GA, Eby KL. Rapid recovery from major depression using magnesium treatment. *Med Hypotheses*. 2006; 67(2):362-70.

Estruch R, Martínez-González MA, Corella D, et al. Effect of a high-fat Mediterranean diet on bodyweight and waist circumference: a prespecified secondary outcomes analysis of the PREDIMED randomised controlled trial. *The Lancet Diabetes & Endocrinology*. 2016. Available from http://www.thelancet.com/journals/landia/article/PIIS2213-8587(16)30085-7/abstract.

Hirayama S, Terasawa K, Rabeler R, et al. The effect of phosphatidylserine administration on memory and symptoms of attention-deficit hyperactivity disorder: a randomised, double-blind, placebo-controlled clinical trial. *J Hum Nutr Diet*. 2014; 27(Suppl 2):284-91.

Itomura M, Hamazaki K, Sawazaki S, et al. The effect of fish oil on physical aggression in schoolchildren – a randomized, double-blind, placebo-controlled trial. *J Nutr Biochem*. 2005; 16(3):163-71.

Jenkins AL, Kacinik V, Lyon MR, et al. Reduction of postprandial glycemia by the novel viscous polysaccharide PGX® in a dose-dependent manner, independent of food form. *J Am Coll Nutr*. 2010; 29(2):92-8.

Kato-Kataoka A, Sakai M, Ebina R, et al. Soybean-derived phosphatidylserine improves memory function of the elderly Japanese subjects with memory complaints. *J Clin Biochem Nutr*. 2010; 47(3):246-55.

Kempton MJ, Ettinger U, Foster R, et al. Dehydration affects brain structure and function in healthy adolescents. Hum Brain Mapp. 2011; 32(1):71-9.

Kidd PM. Phosphatidylserine; membrane nutrient for memory. A clinical and mechanistic assessment. *Altern Med Rev*. 1996; 28:61-6.

Lewis MD, Hibbeln JR, Johnson JE, et al. Suicide deaths of active-duty US military and omega-3 fatty-acid status: a case-control comparison. *J Clin Psychiatry*. 2011; 72(12):1585-90.

Ma T, Tan MS, Yu JT, et al. Resveratrol as a therapeutic agent for Alzheimer's disease. *Biomed Res Int*. 2014; 2014:350-516.

Mardinoglu A, Shoaie S, Bergentall M, et al. The gut microbiota modulates host amino acid and glutathione metabolism in mice. *Molecular Systems Biology*, 2015; 11(10):834.

Noriega BS, Sanchez-Gonzalez MA, Salyakina D, et al. Understanding the impact of omega-3 rich diet on the gut microbiota. *Case Reports in Medicine*. 2016. Available from http://www.hindawi.com/journals/crim/2016/3089303/.

Packer L, Tritschler HJ, Wessel K. Neuroprotection by the metabolic antioxidant alpha-lipoic acid. *Brain Behav*. 1997; 22(1-2):359-78.

Rodriguez-Leyva D, Weighell W, Edel Al, et al. Potent antihypertensive action of dietary flaxseed in hypertensive patients. *Hypertension*. 2013; 62(6):1081-9.

Sanchez-Villegas A, Galbete C, Martinez-Gonzalez MA, et al. The effect of the Mediterranean diet on plasma brain-derived neurotrophic factor (BDNF) levels: the PREDIMED-NAVARRA randomized trial. *Nutr Neurosci*. 2011; 14(5):195-201.

Sawazaki S, Hamazaki T, Yazawa K, et al. The effect of docosahexaenoic acid on plasma catecholamine concentrations and glucose tolerance during long-lasting psychological stress: a double-blind placebo-controlled study. *J Nutr Sci Vitaminol*. (Tokyo). 1999; 45:655-65.

Sublette ME, Hibbeln JR, Galfalvy H, et al. Omega-3 polyunsaturated essential fatty acid status as a predictor of future suicide risk. *Am J Psychiatry*. 2006; 163(6):1100-2.

Tribble, DL. Antioxidant consumption and risk of coronary heart disease: emphasis on vitamin C, vitamin E, and β-carotene. *Circulation*. Section 3. 1999; 99:591-5.

Tzounis X, Rodriguez-Mateos A, Vulevic J, et al. Prebiotic evaluation of cocoa-derived flavanols in healthy humans by using a randomized, controlled, double-blind, cross-over intervention study. *Am J Clin Nutr*. 2011; 93(1):62-72.

Vakhapova V, Richter Y, Cohen T, et al. Safety of phosphatidylserine containing omega-3 fatty acids in non-demented elderly: a double-blind placebo-controlled trial followed by an open-label extension. *BMC Neurology*. 2011; 11:79.

Vuksan V, Sievenpiper JL, Owen R, et al. Beneficial effects of viscous dietary fiber from Konjac-mannan in subjects with the insulin resistance syndrome: results of a controlled metabolic trial. *Diabetes Care*. 2000; 23(1):9-14.

Witte AV, Kerti L, Margulies DS, et al. Effects of resveratrol on memory performance, hippocampal functional connectivity, and glucose metabolism in healthy older adults. *J Neurosci*. 2014; 34(23):7862-70.

Zeisel, SH, da-Costa KA. Choline: an essential nutrient for public health. *Nutr Rev*. 2009; 67(11):615-23.

Chapter 6

American Society for Microbiology. Humans have ten times more bacteria than human cells: how do microbial communities affect human health? *Science Daily*. 2008 June. Available from https://www.sciencedaily.com/releases/2008/06/080603085914.htm.

Arnold LE, Amato A, Bozzolo H, et al. Acetyl-L-carnitine (ALC) in attention-deficit/hyperactivity disorder: a multi-site, placebo-controlled pilot trial. *J Child Adolesc Psychopharmacol*. 2007; 17(6):791-802.

Bélanger SA, Vanasse M, Spahis S, et al. Omega-3 fatty acid treatment of children with attention-deficit hyperactivity disorder: a randomized, double-blind, placebo-controlled study. *Paediatr Child Health*. 2009; 14(2):89-98.

Brault MC, Lacourse E. Prevalence of prescribed attention-deficit hyperactivity disorder medications and diagnosis among Canadian preschoolers and school-age children: 1994-2007. *Can J Psychiatry*. 2012; 57(2):93-101.

Buka I, Osornio-Vargas A, Clark B. Food additives, essential nutrients and neurodevelopmental behavioural disorders in children: a brief review. *Paediatr Child Health*. 2011; 16(7):e54-6.

Burgess RB, Stevens L, Zhang W, et al. Long chain polyunsaturated fatty acids in children with attention-deficit hyperactivity disorder. *Am J Clin Nutr*. 2007; 71(1):327S-305.

Coleman N, Dexhaimer P, DiMascio A, et al. Deanol in the treatment of hyperkinetic children. *Psychosomatics*. 1976; 17(2):68-72.

Currie J, Stabile M, Jones LE. Do stimulant medications improve educational and behavioral outcomes for children with ADHD? Working Paper 19105. *Cambridge: National Bureau of Economic Research*; 2013.

Devaraj S, Vega-Lopez S, Kaul N, et al. Supplementation with a pine bark extract rich in polyphenols increases plasma antioxidant capacity and alters the plasma lipoprotein profile. *Lipids*. 2002; 37(10):931-4.

Dvoráková M, Jezova D, Blazicek P, et al. Urinary catecholamines in children with attention deficit hyperactivity disorder (ADHD): modulation by a polyphenolic extract from pine bark (Pycnogenol). *Nutr Neurosci*. 2007; 10(3-4):151-7.

Dvoráková M, Sivonova M, Trebaticka J, et al. The effect of polyphenolic extract from pine bark, Pycnogenol® on the level of glutathione in children suffering from attention deficit hyperactivity disorder (ADHD). *Redox Rep*. 2006; 11(4):163-72.

Hoza B, Smith AL, Shoulberg EK, et al. A randomized trial examining the effects of aerobic physical activity on attention deficit/hyperactivity disorder symptoms in young children. *J Abnorm Child Psychol*. 2015; 43(4):655-67.

Kheirvari S, Uezu K, Yamamoto S, et al. High-dose dietary supplementation of vitamin A induces brain-derived neurotrophic factor and nerve growth factor production in mice with simultaneous deficiency of vitamin A and zinc. *Nutr Neurosci*. 2008; 11(5):228-34.

Koláček M, Muchova J, Dvorakova M, et al. Effect of natural polyphenols (Pycnogenol) on oxidative stress markers in children suffering from Crohn's disease—a pilot study. *Free Radic Res*. 2013; 47(8):624-34.

Konofal E, Lecendreux M, Deron J, et al. Effects of iron supplementation on attention deficit hyperactivity disorder in children. *Pediatr Neurol*. 2008; 38(1):20-6.

Lewis JA, Young R. Deanol and methylphenidate in minimal brain dysfunction. *Clin Pharmacol Ther*. 1975; 17(5):534-40.

Malitz S, Wilkens B, Higgins JC, et al. A pilot evaluation of deanol in the treatment of anxiety. *Curr Ther Res Clin Exp*. 1967; 9(5):261-4.

Manor I, Magen A, Keidar D, et al. The effect of phosphatidylserine containing omega3 fatty-acids on attention-deficit hyperactivity disorder symptoms in children: a double-blind placebo-controlled trial, followed by an open-label extension. *Eur Psychiatry*. 2012; 27(5):335-42.

McCann D, Barrett A, Cooper A, et al. Food additives and hyperactive behaviours in 3-year-old and 8/9-year-old children in the community: a randomized double-blinded placebo controlled trial. *Lancet*. 2007; 370(9598):1560-7.

Morrow RL, Garland EJ, Wright JM, et al. Influence of relative age on diagnosis and treatment of attention-deficit/hyperactivity disorder in children. *CMAJ*. 2012; 184(7):755-62.

Morton WA, Stockton GG. Methylphenidate abuse and psychiatric side effects. *J Clin Psychiatry*. 2000; 2(5):159-64.

Niederhofer H. Association of attention-deficit/hyperactivity disorder and celiac disease: a brief report. *Prim Care Companion CNS Disord*. 2011; 13(3):PCC.10br01104.

Pfeiffer , CC, Jenney EH, Gallagher W, et al. Stimulant effect of 2-dimethyl-1-aminoethanol: possible precursor of brain acetylcholine. *Science*. 1957; 126:610-1.

Raz R, Gabis L. Essential fatty acids and attention-deficit-hyperactivity disorder: a systematic review. *Dev Med Child Neurol*. 2009; 51(8):580-92.

Richardson, AJ. Clinical trials of fatty acid treatment in ADHD, dyslexia, dyspraxia and the autistic spectrum. *Prostaglandins Leukot Essent Fatty Acids*. 2004 ; 70(4):383-90.

Richardson AJ, Montgomery P. The Oxford-Durham study: a randomized, controlled trial of dietary supplementation with fatty acids in children with developmental coordination disorder. *Pediatrics*. 2005; 115(5):1360-6.

Shin JY, Roughead EE, Byung-Joo Park BJ, et al. Cardiovascular safety of methylphenidate among children and young people with attention-deficit/hyperactivity disorder (ADHD): nationwide self controlled case series study. *Brit Med J.* 2016; 353:i2550.

Trebatická J, Kopasova S, Hradecna Z, et al. Treatment of ADHD with French maritime pine bark extract, Pycnogenol. *Eur Child Adolesc Psychiatry.* 2006; 15(6): 329-35.

US Department of Justice. *Methylphenidate* (a background paper). National Criminal Justice Reference Service. 1995. Available from https://www.ncjrs.gov/App/Publications/abstract.aspx?ID=163349.

Volkow, ND, Ding Y-S, Fowler JS, et al. Is methylphenidate like cocaine? Studies on their pharmacokinetics and distribution in the human brain. *JAMA Psychiatry.* 1995; 52(6):456-63.

Wagner-Schuman M. Richardson JR, Auinger P, et al. Association of pyrethroid pesticide exposure with attention-deficit/hyperactivity disorder in a nationally representative sample of U.S. children. *Environmental Health.* 2015; 14(44):1-9.

SECTION 4
Chapter 7

Abdou AM, Higashiguchi S, Horie K, et al. Relaxation and immunity enhancement effects of gamma-aminobutyric acid (GABA) administration in humans. *BioFactors.* 2006; 26(3):201-8.

Adams PW, Wynn V, Rose DP, et al. Effect of pyridoxine hydrochloride (vitamin B6) upon depression associated with oral contraception. *Lancet.* 1973; 201(7809):897-904.

Akhondzadeh S, Fallah-Pour H, Afkham K, et al. Comparison of *Crocus sativus* L. and imipramine in the treatment of mild to moderate depression: a pilot double-blind randomized trial. *BMC Complement Altern Med.* 2004; 4(12):1-5.

Akhondzadeh S, Tahmacebi-Pour N, Noorbala A-A, et al. *Crocus sativus* L. in the treatment of mild to moderate depression: a double-blind, randomized and placebo-controlled trial. *Phytother Res.* 2005; 19(2):148-151.

Anderson RA, Polansky MM, Brydan NA, et al. Effects of supplemental chromium on patients with symptoms of reactive hypoglycemia. *Metabolism.* 1987; 36(4):351-5.

Avena NE, Rada P, Hoebel BG. Evidence for sugar addiction: behavioral and neurochemical effects of intermittent, excessive sugar intake. *Neurosci Biobehav Rev.* 2008:31(1):20-39.

Beckmann H, Athen D, Olteanu M, et al. dl-Phenylalanine versus imipramine: a double-blind controlled study. *Eur Arch Psychiatry Clin Neurosci.* 1979; 227(1):49-58.

Beckmann H, Ludolph E. DL-phenylalanine as an antidepressant. Open study. *Arzneimittel-Forschung.* 1978; 28(8):1283-4.

Bell IR, Edman JS, Morrow FD, et al. B complex vitamin patterns in geriatric and young adult inpatients with major depression. *J Am Geriatr Soc.* 1991; 39(3):252-7.

Bottiglieri T. Folate, vitamin B12, and neuropsychiatric disorders. *Nutr Rev.* 1996; 54(12):382-90.

Brodie HKH, Sack R, Siever L. Clinical studies of L-5-hydroxytryptophan in depression. In: Barchas J and Usdin E, editors. *Serotonin and behavior.* New York: Academic Press; 1973.

Buydens-Branchey L, Branchey M, Hibbeln JR. Associations between increases in plasma n-3 polyunsaturated fatty acids following supplementation and decreases in anger and anxiety in substance abusers. *Prog Neuropsychopharmacol Biol Psychiatry.* 2008; 32(2):568-75.

Byerley WF, Judd LL, Reimherr FW, et al. 5-hydroxytryptophan: a review of its antidepressant efficacy and adverse effects. *J Clin Psychopharmacol.* 1987; 7(3):127-37.

Chandrasekhar KA. Prospective, randomized double-blind, placebo-controlled study of safety and efficacy of a high-concentration full-spectrum extract of Ashwagandha root in reducing stress and anxiety in adults. *Indian J Psychol Med.* 2012; 34(3):255-62.

Chih-chiang, C, Peilun Liu J, Su K-P. The use of omega-3 fatty acids in treatment of depression. *Psychiatric Times.* 2008; 25(9):76-80.

Coppen A, Bolander-Gouaille C. Treatment of depression: time to consider folic acid and vitamin B12. *J Psychopharmacol.* 2005; 19(1):59-65.

Eschenauer G, Sweet BV. Pharmacology and therapeutic uses of theanine. *Am J Health Syst Pharm.* 2006; 63(1):28-30.

Fournier JC, DeRubeis RJ, Hollon SD, et al. Antidepressant drug effects and depression severity: a patient-level meta-analysis. *JAMA.* 2010; 303(1):47-53.

Freeman MP, Rapaport MH. Omega-3 fatty acids and depression: from cellular mechanisms to clinical care. *J Clin Psychiatry.* 2011; 72(2):258-9.

Gilbody S, Lightfoot T, Sheldon T. Is low folate a risk factor for depression? A meta-analysis and exploration of heterogeneity. *J Epidemiol Community Health.* 2007; 61:631-7.

Goggans, FC. A case of mania secondary to vitamin B12 deficiency. Am J Psychiatry. 1984; 141(2):300-1.

Hasanah CI, Khan UA, Musalmah M, et al. Reduced red-cell folate in mania. *J Affect Disord.* 1997; 46(2):95-9.

Hasler G, vander Veen JW, Tumonins T, et al. Reduced prefrontal glutamate/glutamine and gamma-aminobutyric acid levels in major depression determined using proton magnetic resonance spectroscopy. *JAMA Psychiatry.* 2007; 64(2):193-200.

Hertz, L, Kvamme E, McGeer EG, et al., editors. *Glutamine, glutamate, and GABA in the central nervous system.* New York: Alan R Liss Inc.; 1983.

Hoes MJ. L-tryptophan in depression and strain. *J Orthomol Med.* 1982; 11(4):231-42.

Kale A, Naphade N, Sapkale S, et al. Reduced folic acid, vitamin B12 and docosahexaenoic acid and increased homocysteine and cortisol in never-medicated schizophrenia patients: implications for altered one-carbon metabolism. *Psychiatry Res.* 2010; 175(1-2):47-53.

Kerr, DCR, Zava Dt, Piper WT, et al. Associations between vitamin D levels and depressive symptoms in healthy young adult women. *Psychiatry Res.* 2015; 227(1):46-51.

Kiecolt-Glasera JK, Belury MA, Andridge R, et al. Omega-3 supplementation lowers inflammation and anxiety in medical students: a randomized controlled trial. *Brain, Behav Immun.* 2011; 25(8):1725-34.

Lakhan SE, Vierira KF. Nutritional therapies for mental disorders. *Nutrition Journal.* 2008; 7(2):1-8.

Lenze EJ, Mantella RC, Shi P, et al. Elevated cortisol in older adults with generalized anxiety disorder is reduced by treatment: a placebo-controlled evaluation of escitalopram. *Am J Geriatr Psychiatry.* 2011; 19(5):482-90.

Leonard BE. The role of noradrenaline in depression: a review. *J Psychopharmacol.* 1997; 11(4):S39-47.

Levine J, Barak Y, Gonzalves M, et al. Double-blind, controlled trial of inositol treatment of depression. *Am J Psychiatry.* 1995; 152(5):792-4.

Lichtman JH, Biggrt JT, Blumenthal, JA. Depression and coronary heart disease. *Circulation.* 2008; 118:1768-75.

Logan, AC. Omega-3 fatty acids and major depression: a primer for the mental health professional. *Lipids Health Dis.* 2004; 3:25.

Lopresti AL, Hood SD, Drummond PD. Multiple antidepressant potential modes of action of curcumin: a review of its anti-inflammatory, monoaminergic, antioxidant, immune-modulating and neuroprotective effects. *J Psychopharmacol.* 2012; 26(12):1512-24.

Lopresti AL, Maes M, Meddens MJM, et al. Curcumin and major depression: a randomised, double-blind, placebo-controlled trial investigating the potential of peripheral biomarkers to predict treatment response and antidepressant mechanisms of change. *Eur Neuropsychopharmacol.* 2015; 25(1):38-50.

McLean A, Rubinsztein JS, Robbins TW, et al. The effects of tyrosine depletion in normal healthy volunteers: implications for unipolar depression. *Psychopharmacol.* 2004; 171(3):286-97.

Merete C, Falcon LM, Tucker KL. Vitamin B6 is associated with depressive symptomatology in Massachusetts elders. *J Am Coll Nutr.* 2008; 27(3):421-7.

Moller HJ. Is there evidence for negative effects of antidepressants on suicidality in depressive patients? A systematic review. *Eur Arch Psychiatry Clin Neurosci.* 2006; 256(8):476-96.

Mukai T, Kishi T, Matsuda Y, et al. A meta-analysis of inositol for depression and anxiety disorders. *Hum Psychopharmacol.* 2014; 29(1):55-63.

Nieper HA. The clinical applications of lithium orotate. A two years study. *Agressologie.* 1973; 14(6):407-11.

Noorbala AA, Akhondzadeh S, Tamacebi-Pour N, et al. Hydro-alcoholic extract of *Crocus sativus* L. versus fluoxetine in the treatment of mild to moderate depression: a double-blind, randomized pilot trial. *J Ethnopharmacol.* 2005; 97:281-4.

O'Donnell T, Rotzinger S, Ulrich M, et al. Effects of chronic lithium and sodium valproate on concentrations of brain amino acids. *Eur Neuropsychopharmacol.* 2003; 13(4):220-7.

Oken RJ. Obsessive-compulsive disorder: a neuronal membrane phospholipid hypothesis and concomitant therapeutic strategy. *Med Hypotheses.* 2001; 56(4):413-5.

Osher Y, Bersudsky Y, Belmaker RH. Omega-3 eicosapentaenoic acid in bipolar depression: report of a small open-label study. *J Clin Psychiatry.* 2005; 66(6):726-9.

Petty F. GABA and mood disorders: a brief review and hypothesis. *J Affect Disord.* 1995; 34(4):275-81.

Rösche J, Uhlmann C, Froscher W. Low serum folate levels as a risk factor for depressive mood in patients with chronic epilepsy. *J Neuropsychiatry Clin Neurosci.* 2003; 15(1):64-6.

Rot M, Moskowitz DS, Pinard G, et al. Social behaviour and mood in everyday life: the effects of tryptophan in quarrelsome individuals. *J Psychiatry Neurosci.* 2006; 31(4):253-62.

Russell AL, McCarty MF. DL-phenylalanine markedly potentiates opiate analgesia – an example of nutrient/pharmaceutical up-regulation of the endogenous analgesic system. *Med Hypotheses.* 2000; 55(4):283-8.

Sartori HE. Lithium orotate in the treatment of alcoholism and related conditions. *Alcohol.* 1986; 3(2):97-100.

Scholey AB, French SJ, Morris PJ, et al. Consumption of cocoa flavanols results in acute improvements in mood and cognitive performance during sustained mental effort. *J Psychopharmacol.* 2010; 24(10):1505-14.

Setiawan E, Wilson AA, Mizrahi R, et al. Role of translocator protein density, a marker of neuroinflammation, in the brain during major depressive episodes. *JAMA Psychiatry.* 2015; 72(3):268-75.

Skarupski KA, Tangney C, Li H, et al. Longitudinal association of vitamin B-6, folate, and vitamin B-12 with depressive symptoms among older adults over time. *Am J Clin Nutr.* 2010; 92(2):330-5.

Stetler C, Miller GE. Blunted cortisol response to awakening in mild to moderate depression: regulatory influences of sleep patterns and social contacts. *J Abnorm Psychol.* 2005; 114(4):697-705.

Tombaugh, TC, Yang SH, Swanson RA, et al. Glucocorticoids exacerbate hypoxic and hypoglycemic hippocampal injury in vitro: biochemical correlates and a role for astrocytes. *J Neurochem.* 1992; 59(1):137-46.

VanPraag HM, Korf F. 5-hydroxytryptophan as antidepressant: the predictive value of the probenecid test. *Psychopharmacol Bull.* 1972; 8:34-5.

Volz, HP, Kieser, M. Kava-kava extract WS 1490 versus placebo in anxiety disorders: a randomized placebo-controlled 25-week outpatient trial. *Pharmacopsychiat.* 1997; 30(1):1-5.

Vreeburg, SA, Witte JG, Hoogendijk RH, et al. Salivary cortisol levels and the 2-year course of depressive and anxiety disorders. *Psychoneuroendocrinology.* 2013; 38(9):1494-502.

Watson AW, Haskell-Ramsay CF, Kennedy DO, et al. Acute supplementation with blackcurrant extracts modulates cognitive functioning and inhibits monoamine oxidase-B in healthy young adults. *J Funct Foods.* 2015; 17:524-39.

REFERENCES

Welbourne TC. Increased plasma bicarbonate and growth hormone after an oral glutamine load. *Am J Clin Nutr.* 1995; 61(5):1058-61.

Wium-Andersen MK, Orsten DD, Nielsen SF, et al. Elevated C-reactive protein levels, psychological distress, and depression in 73,131 individuals. *JAMA Psychiatry.* 2013; 70(2):1-9.

Young LS, Bye R, Scheltinga M, et al. Patients receiving glutamine-supplemented intravenous feedings report an improvement in mood. *J Parenter Enteral Nutr.* 1993; 17(5):422-7.

Young SN. Folate and depression – a neglected problem. *J Psychiatry Neurosci.* 2007; 32(2):80-2.

Chapter 8

Aguirre-Hernandez E, Martinez AL, Gonzalez-Trujano ME, et al. Pharmacological evaluation of the anxiolytic and sedative effects of Tilia americana L. var. mexicana in mice. *J Ethnopharmacol.* 2007; 109(1):140-5.

Akhondzadeh S, Naghavi HR, Vazirian M, et al. Passionflower in the treatment of generalized anxiety: a pilot double-blind randomized controlled trial with oxazepam. *J Clin Pharm Ther.* 2001 Oct; 26(5):363-7.

Appel K, Rose T, Fiebich B, et al. Modulation of the γ-aminobutyric acid (GABA) system by *Passiflora incarnata* L. *Phytother Res.* 2011 Jun; 25(6):838-43.

Balbo M, Leproult R, Van Cauter E. Impact of sleep and its disturbances on hypothalamo-pituitary-adrenal axis activity. *Int J Endocrinol.* 2010; 2010:1-16.

Basta M, Chrousos GP, Vela-Bueno A, et al. Chronic insomnia and stress system. *Sleep Med Clin.* 2007; 2(2):279-91.

Blumenthal M, Goldberg A, Brinckmann J. *Herbal medicine: expanded Commission E monographs.* Newton, MA: Integrative Medicine Communications; 2000.

Brown E, Hurd NS, McCall S, et al. Evaluation of the anxiolytic effects of chrysin, a *Passiflora incarnata* extract, in the laboratory rat. *AANA J.* 2007 Oct; 75(5):333-7.

Buscemi N, Vandermeer B, Pandya R, et al. Melatonin for treatment of sleep disorders: summary. *Agency for Healthcare Research and Quality.* Publication Number 05-E002-1. 2004. Available from http://archive.ahrq.gov/clinic/epcsums/melatsum.htm.

Cauffield JS, Forbes HJ. Dietary supplements used in the treatment of depression, anxiety, and sleep disorders. *Lippincotts Prim Care Pract.* 1999; 3:290-304.

Coleta M, Campos MG, Cotrin MD, et al. Comparative evaluation of *Melissa officinalis* L., *Tilia eruopaea* L., *Passiflora edulis* Sims. and *Hypericum perforatum* L. in the elevated plus maze anxiety test. *Pharmacopsychiatry.* 2001; 34 Suppl 1:S20-1.

Dhawan K, Dhawan S, Chhabra S. Attenuation of benzodiazepine dependence in mice by a tri-substituted benzoflavone moiety of *Passiflora incarnata* Linneaus: A non-habit forming anxiolytic. *J Pharm Pharmaceut Sci.* 2003; 6(2):215–22.

Dominguez RA, Bravo-Valverde RL, Kaplowitz BR, et al.

Valerian as a hypnotic for Hispanic patients. *Cult Divers Ethinic Minor Psychol.* 2000; 6(1):84-92.

Elsas SM, Rossi DJ, Rabera J, et al. *Passiflora incarnata* L. (Passionflower) extracts elicit GABA currents in hippocampal neurons in vitro, and show anxiogenic and anticonvulsant effects in vivo, varying with extraction-method. *Phytomedicine.* 2010 October; 17(12):940–9.

Gafner S, Dietz BM, McPhail KL, et al. Alkaloids from *Eschscholzia californica* and their capacity to inhibit binding of [3H]8-Hydroxy-2-(di-N-propylamino)tetralin to 5-HT1A receptors in Vitro. *J Nat Prod.* 2006; 69(3):432-5.

Gottesmann C. GABA mechanisms and sleep. *Neuroscience.* 2002; 111(2):231-9.

Hanus M, Lafon J, Mathieu M. Double-blind, randomised, placebo-controlled study to evaluate the efficacy and safety of a fixed combination containing two plant extracts (*Crataegus oxyacantha* and *Eschscholtzia californica*) and magnesium in mild-to-moderate anxiety disorders. *Curr Med Res Opin.* 2004; 20:63-71.

Lewis JG. Steroid analysis in saliva: an overview. *Clin Biochem Rev.* 2006; 27(3):139-46.

Medina JH, Viola H, Wolfman C, et al. Flavonoids: a new family of benzodiazepine receptor ligands. *Neurochem Res.* 1997; 22:419-25.

National institutes of health office of dietary supplements. *Valerian: fact sheet for health professionals.* March 2013. Available from https://ods.od.nih.gov/factsheets/Valerian-HealthProfessional/.

Ngan A, Conduit R. A double-blind, placebo-controlled investigation of the effects of *Passiflora incarnate* (passionflower) herbal tea on subjective sleep quality. *Phytother Res.* 2011 Aug; 25(8):1153-9.

Pérez-Ortega G, Guevara-Fefer P, Chávez M, et al. Sedative and anxiolytic efficacy of *Tilia americana* var. mexicana inflorescences used traditionally by communities of State of Michoacan, Mexico. *J Ethnopharmacol.* 2008 Mar 28; 116(3):461-8.

Rolland A, Fleurentin J, Lanhers MC, et al. Behavioural effects of the American traditional plant *Eschscholzia californica*: sedative and anxiolytic properties. *Planta Med.* 1991; 57:212-6.

Rolland A, Fleurentin J, Lanhers MC, et al. Neurophysiological effects of an extract of *Eschscholzia californica* Cham. (Papaveraceae). *Phytother Res.* 2001; 15:377-81.

Shinomiya K, Inoue T, Utsu Y, et al. Hypnotic activities of chamomile and passiflora extracts in sleepdisturbed rats. *Biol Pharm Bull.* 2005 May; 28(5):808-10.

Soulairac A, Lambinet H. Effect of 5-hydroxytryptophan, a serotonin precursor, on sleep disorders. *Ann Med Psychol.* 1977; 1(5):792-8.

Törnhage CJ. Salivary cortisol for assessment of hypothalamic-pituitary-adrenal axis function. *Neuroimmunomodulation.* 2009; 16(5):284-9.

Van Cauter E, Knutson K, Leproult R, et al. The impact of sleep deprivation on hormones and metabolism. *Neurology.*

2005; 7(1). Available from http://www.medscape.org/viewarticle/502825.

Wad R, Arnason JT, Trudeau V, et al. Phytochemical and biological analysis of skullcap (*Scutellaria lateriflora* L.): a medicinal plant with anxiolytic properties. *Phytomedicine.* 2003; 10:640-9.

Wolfson P, Hoffmann DL. An investigation into the efficacy of *Scutellaria lateriflora* in healthy volunteers. *Altern Ther Health Med.* 2003; 9:74-8.

Zhdanova IV, Wurtman RJ, Regan MM, et al. Melatonin treatment for age-related insomnia. *J Clin Endocrinol Metab.* 2001; 86(10):4727-30.

Ziegler G, Ploch M, Miettinen-Baumann A, et al. Efficacy and tolerability of valerian extract LI 156 compared with oxazepam in the treatment of non-organic insomnia – a randomized, double-blind, comparative clinical study. *Eur J Med Res.* 2002; 7(11):480-6.

Chapter 9

Arnsten, AFT. Stress signalling pathways that impair prefrontal cortex structure and function. *Nat Rev Neurosci.* 2009; 10:410-22.

Balestreri R, Fontana L, Astengo F. A double-blind placebo controlled evaluation of the safety and efficacy of vinpocetine in the treatment of patients with chronic vascular senile cerebral dysfunction. *J Am Geriatr Soc.* 1987; 35(5):425-30.

Barcelos RCS, Benvegnu DM, Boufleur N, et al. Effects of omega-3 essential fatty acids (omega-3 EFAs) on motor disorders and memory dysfunction typical neuroleptic-induced: behavioral and biochemical parameter. *Neurotox Res.* 2010; 17(3):228-37.

Bavarsad Shahripour R, Harrigan MR, Alexandrov AV. N-acetylcysteine (NAC) in neurological disorders: mechanisms of action and therapeutic opportunities. *Brain Behav.* 2014; 4(2):108-22.

Bégin ME, Langlois MF, Lorrain D, et al. Thyroid function and cognition during aging. *Curr Gerontol Geriatr Res.* 2008; 2008:1-11.

Bremner JD. Traumatic stress: effects on the brain. *Dialogues Clin Neurosci.* 2006; 8(4):445-61.

Brüning JC, Gautam D, Burks DJ, et al. Role of brain insulin receptor in control of body weight and reproduction. *Science.* 2000; 289(5487):2122-5.

Collet T-H, Gussekloo J, Bauer DC, et al. Subclinical hyperthyroidism and the risk of coronary heart disease and mortality. *JAMA Internal Medicine.* 2012; 172(10):799-809.

Conrad CD. Chronic stress-induced hippocampal vulnerability: the glucocorticoid vulnerability hypothesis. *Rev Neurosci.* 2008; 19(6):395-412.

Cooper C, Sommerlad A, Lyketsos CG, et al. Modifiable predictors of dementia in mild cognitive impairment: a systematic review and meta-analysis. *Am J Psychiatry.* 2015; 172(4):323-34.

Davison K, Berry NM, Misan G, et al. Dose-related effects of flavanol-rich cocoa on blood pressure. *J Hum Hypertens.*

2010; 24(9):568-76.

De Jager CA, Oulhaj A, Jacoby R, et al. Cognitive and clinical outcomes of homocysteine-lowering B-vitamin treatment in mild cognitive impairment: a randomized controlled trial. *Int J Geriatr Psychiatry.* 2012 Jun; 27(6):592-600.

Dean O, Giorlando F, Berk M. N-acetylcysteine in psychiatry: current therapeutic evidence and potential mechanisms of action. *J Psychiatry Neurosci.* 2011; 36(2):78-86.

Desideri G, Kwik-Uribe C, Grassi D, et al. Benefits in cognitive function, blood pressure, and insulin resistance through cocoa flavanol consumption in elderly subjects with mild cognitive impairment: the Cocoa, Cognition, and Aging (CoCoA) Study. *Hypertension.* 2012; 60:794-801.

Dobos N, Korf J, Luiten PG, et al. Neuroinflammation in Alzheimer's disease and major depression. *J Psyc Neuroscience.* 2010; 67(6):503-4.

Dong H, Csernansky JG. Effects of stress and stress hormones on amyloid-β protein and plaque deposition. *J Alzheimers Dis.* 2009; 18(2):459-69.

Farr SA, Poon HF, Dogrukol-Ak D, et al. The antioxidants alpha-lipoic acid and N-acetylcysteine reverse memory impairment and brain oxidative stress in aged SAMP8 mice. *J Neurochem.* 2003; 84:1173-83.

Feher G, Koltai K, Kesmarky G, et al. Effect of parenteral or oral vinpocetine on the hemorheological parameters of patients with chronic cerebrovascular diseases. *Phytomedicine.* 2009; 16(1-2):111-7.

Figlewicz DP, Szot P, Chavez M, et al. Intraventricular insulin increases dopamine transporter mRNA in rat VTA/substantia nigra. *Brain Res.* 1994; 644(2):331-4.

Havrankova J, Roth J, Brownstein M. Insulin receptors are widely distributed in the central nervous system of the rat. *Nature.* 1978; 272:827-9.

Javed H, Khan A, Vaibhav K, et al. Taurine ameliorates neurobehavioral, neurochemical and immunohistochemical changes in sporadic dementia of Alzheimer's type (SDAT) caused by intracerebroventricular streptozotocin in rats. *Neurol Sci.* 2013; 34(12):2181-92.

Jerneren F, Elshorbagy AK, Oulhaj A, et al. Brain atrophy in cognitively impaired elderly: the importance of long-chain omega-3 fatty acids and B vitamin status in a randomized controlled trial. *Am J Clin Nutr.* 2015; 102:215-2.

Kanai M, Otsuka Y, Otsuka K, et al. A phase I study investigating the safety and pharmacokinetics of highly bioavailable curcumin (Theracurmin) in cancer patients. *Cancer Chemother Pharmacol.* 2013; 71(6):1521-30.

Kemény V, Molnar S, Andrejkovics M, et al. Acute and chronic effects of vinpocetine on cerebral hemodynamics and neuropsychological performance in multi-infarct patients. *J Clin Pharmacol.* 2005; 45(9):1048-54.

Kobayashi S, Iwamoto M, Kon K, et al. Acetyl-L-carnitine improves aged brain function. *Geriatr Gerontol Int.* 2010; 10(s1):S99-S106.

REFERENCES

Koch, S. Walking backwards may sharpen thinking. *Psychol Sci.* 2009; 20:549-50.

Könner AC, Hess S, Tovar S, et al. Role for insulin signaling in catecholaminergic neurons in control of energy homeostasis. *Cell Metab.* 2011; 13(6):720-8.

Lonskaya I, Hebron M, Chen W, et al. Tau deletion impairs intra cellular β-amyloid-42 clearance and leads to more extracellular plaque deposition in gene transfer models. *Mol Neurodegener.* 2014; 9:46.

Lou HC. Dopamine precursors and brain function in phenylalanine hydroxylase deficiency. *Acta Paediatr Suppl.* 1994; 83(s407):86-8.

Louzada PR, Lima ACP, Mendonca-Silva DL, et al. Taurine prevents the neurotoxicity of beta-amyloid and glutamate receptor agonists: activation of GABA receptors and possible implications for Alzheimer's disease and other neurological disorders. *FASEB J.* 2004; 18(3):511-8.

Lupien SJ, de Leon M, de Santi S, et al. Cortisol levels during human aging predict hippocampal atrophy and memory deficits. *Nat Neurosci.* 1998; 1:69-73.

Moretti R, Torre P, Antonello RM, et al. Risk factors for vascular dementia: hypotension as a key point. *Vasc Health Risk Manag.* 2008; 4(2):395-402.

Ng TP, Chiam P-C, Lee T, et al. Curry consumption and cognitive function the elderly. *Am J Epidemiol.* 2006; 164(9):898-906.

Nussbaum JM, Schilling S, Cynis H, et al. Prion-like behaviour and tau-dependent cytotoxicity of pyroglutamylated amyloid-⊠. Nature. 2012; 485(7400):651-5.

Ohwada K, Takeda H, Yamazaki M, et al. Pyrroloquinoline quinone (PQQ) prevents cognitive deficit caused by oxidative stress in rats. *J Clin Biochem Nutr.* 2008; 42(1):29-34.

Pase MP, Scholey AB, Pipingas A, et al. Cocoa polyphenols enhance positive mood states but not cognitive performance: a randomized, placebo-controlled trial. *J Psychopharmacol.* 2013; 27(5):451-8.

Sabaratnam V, Kah-Hui W, Naidu M, et al. Neuronal health – can culinary and medicinal mushrooms help? *J Tradit Complement Med.* 2013; 3(1):62-8.

Scholey AB, French SJ, Morris PJ, et al. Consumption of cocoa flavanols results in acute improvements in mood and cognitive performance during sustained mental effort. *J Psychopharmacol.* 2010; 24(10):1505-14.

Sen A, Heaton J, Whiley L. Evidence of altered phosphatidylcholine metabolism in Alzheimer's disease. *Neurobiol Aging.* 2014; 35:271-8.

Shrikant M, Palanivelu K. The effect of curcumin (turmeric) on Alzheimer's disease: an overview. *Ann Indian Acad Neurol.* 2008; 11(1):13-9.

Sun QQ, Xu SS, Pan JL, et al. Huperzine-A capsules enhance memory and learning performance in 34 pairs of matched adolescent students. *Zhongguo Yao Li Xue Bao.* 1999; 20(7):601-3.

Szilágyi G, Nazy Z, Balkay L, et al. Effects of vinpocetine on the redistribution of cerebral blood flow and glucose metabolism in chronic ischemic stroke patients: a PET study. *J Neurol Sci.* 2005; 229-230:275-84.

Tan ZS, Beiser A, Vasan RS, et al. Thyroid function and the risk of Alzheimer's disease. *Arch Intern Med.* 2008; 168(14):1514-20.

Tzounis X, Rodriguez-Mateos A, Vulevic J, et al. Prebiotic evaluation of cocoa-derived flavanols in healthy humans by using a randomized, controlled, double-blind, crossover intervention study. *Am J Clin Nutr.* 2011; 93(1):62-72.

Witte AV, Kerti L, Hermannstandter HM, et al. Long-chain omega-3 fatty acids improve brain function and structure in older adults. *Cereb Cortex.* 2014 Nov; 24(11):3059-68.

Xiao Z, Zhang A, Lin J, et al. Telomerase: a target for therapeutic effects of curcumin and a curcumin derivative in aβ1-42 insult in vitro. *PLoS One.* 2014; 9(7):e101251.

Xie H, Wang J-R, Yau L-F, et al. Catechins and procyanidins of *Ginkgo biloba* show potent activities towards the inhibition of β-amyloid peptide aggregation and destabilization of preformed fibrils. *Molecules.* 2014; 19(4):5119-34.

Xu Z-Q, Ling X-M, Juan-Wu L, et al. Treatment with huperzine A improves cognition in vascular dementia patients. *Cell Biochem Biophys.* 2012; 62(1):55-8.

Yang G, Want Y, Tian J, et al. Huperzine A for Alzheimer's disease: a systematic review and meta-analysis of randomized clinical trials. *PLoS One.* 2013; 8(9):e74916.

Yarchoan M, Arnold SE. Repurposing diabetes drugs for brain insulin resistance in Alzheimer disease. *Diabetes.* 2014; 63(7):2253-61.

Zandi PP, Anthony JC, Khachaturian AS, et al. Reduced risk of Alzheimer disease in users of antioxidant vitamin supplements: the Cache County Study. *Arch Neurol.* 2004; 61(1):82-8.

Zhang L, Fiala M, Cashman J, et al. Curcuminoids enhance amyloid-beta uptake by macrophages of Alzheimer's disease patients. *J Alzheimers Dis.* 2006; 10:1-7.

At A Glance – The Optimal Use Guide

At A Glance provides an overview of supplements and suggestions to help attain and maintain optimal brain health, as well as prevention and recovery tips for many common mental health disorders. The main text of the book provides more detail on each condition, the science and research proving the benefits of using natural remedies, and the influence of the three brains on mental and emotional well-being.

Optimal You

The human brain is a mysterious 1.4 kg (3 lb) organ that controls, integrates, and interprets information from the outside world through the five senses. Or so we thought! Recent research has found we actually have three brains: the heart, gut, and head brains. The three brains work together to influence who we are and how we interact with the world around us.

The Gut-Brain Axis

The head brain has about 100 billion neurons. The gut brain has close to 500 million nerve cells and 100 million neurons and is about the size of a cat's brain. The gut brain works independently and in conjunction with the head brain.

In recent years gut microbiota has become a major topic of research. Studies are now revealing how variations in the composition of gut microbiota contribute to diseases ranging from inflammation to obesity, as well as mental health disorders including cognitive problems, anxiety, and depression and other mood disorders.

Biologists at the University of California, San Diego, have discovered that bacteria, often viewed as lowly little creatures, are actually quite sophisticated in their social interactions. In fact, they communicate with one another through similar electrical signalling mechanisms as neurons in the head brain.

The emerging concept of a gut-brain axis suggests that modulation of gut microbiota with probiotics, which introduce good bacteria into the gut, may be a new approach for the treatment of some mental health and neurological disorders. Although probiotics won't be replacing antidepressants anytime soon, they are a very important part of any health program.

The Heart-Brain Axis

Scientists initially became interested in the heart-brain connection because of the personality changes observed in heart transplant patients. Some recipients took on more of the characteristics and personality of the person who donated the heart. This has led to more research on the heart-brain connection.

Until the 1990s, scientists assumed, and most of us were taught, that only the brain sent information and issued commands to the heart and the rest of the body. Now we know that the heart brain is an intricate network of approximately 40,000 neurons and other support cells that help us sense, feel, learn, and remember.

Roles of the Three Brains

Apart from the obvious different physical functions of each organ, the head, heart, and gut brains also perform different mental and emotional functions. For example, the head brain is used for analyzing information and applying logic. The heart brain senses the world through emotion and feelings, and the gut helps us learn self-preservation by teaching us to follow our instinct – the "gut feeling" we all experience at times.

When people feel "normal", they interact with others and the world around them in their own unique way and this interaction becomes part of their identity. As mentioned in the introduction, all health problems and disease conditions bring pain and suffering of various degrees and in different ways, but brain disorders are the only conditions that change, distort, or in some cases rob people of their "essence", their identity – who they are in the world.

How to Attain and Maintain the "Optimal You"

Maintaining optimal function of the three brains is crucial to being the best you can be – the optimal you. Life today presents many challenges that can interfere with this state of being. What can you do to maintain optimal function of the three brains?

Eating for the Optimal You

Fuel for the three brains starts with a good diet and lifestyle and added supplements to provide the necessary building blocks. Carbohydrates are required for energy; proteins for the synthesis of the chemical messengers, the neurotransmitters in the three brains; antioxidants to prevent free radical damage and inflammation; and good fats to build and protect neurons in the three brains. Water is the often-forgotten nutrient and it is critical for healthy brains.

The Mediterranean diet is an excellent dietary guide to follow to maintain healthy three-brain function, along with drinking at least 1.5 litres of water a day. The brain is 73% water and a dehydrated shriveled brain does not perform well. Super foods provide extra levels of antioxidants and nutrients for optimal three-brain function. (Refer to Chapter 5 for more information on diet and lifestyle for three-brain health.)

It is also important to address factors that can interfere with optimal brain function, including food allergies, inflammation, blood sugar imbalances, gut microbiota, and environmental toxins. Addressing these factors can be a very potent and effective treatment for many people with mental health disorders, without the risk of side effects.

Different protective networks are in place to protect the three brains from coming in contact with most toxins and infectious agents. However, several factors can break down the defensive systems, including high blood pressure, inflammation, environmental toxins, stress hormones, heavy metals, gut microbes, medications, and food allergies, to name a few. The following suggestions are ways to help reduce the impact of these "brain busters":

- Reduce inflammation
- Balance metabolism and control blood sugar levels
- Maintain a healthy gut microbiota (gut-brain axis)
- Remember the importance of the heart-brain connection
- Eliminate food allergies and food intolerances
- Avoid gluten if you are gluten sensitive or intolerant
- Avoid GMO foods
- Eliminate trans fats
- Minimize exposure to electromagnetic frequencies (EMFs)
- Be aware of and minimize exposure to environmental toxins and heavy metals

- Reduce sugar and refined carbohydrate intake
- Understand the negative effects of prescription medicine on the three brains

(Refer to Chapters 3 and 4 for more information about brain busters and how to reduce their impact.)

Scientific evidence shows that nutritional supplementation helps control symptoms of mental health disorders including depression, bipolar disorder, schizophrenia, anxiety disorders, cognitive and learning disorders, and addictions. The general population in North America is often deficient in vitamins, minerals, and omega-3 fatty acids, and individuals suffering from mental health disorders are often exceptionally deficient.

> A growing number of consumers are choosing natural health products as a legitimate and sound healthcare option. However, not all supplements are created equal. For added confidence in the quality and safety of products, look for ISURA™-certified supplements. Natural health products that have passed a battery of laboratory tests are granted the ISURA seal of approval, which guarantees that the products are safe, uncontaminated, of high quality, of guaranteed potency, GMO-free, and properly labelled. For more information, go to www.isura.ca.

Supplement Support for the Three Brains

In today's modern world we are encouraged to focus mainly on listening to our head brain. But we also need to learn to recognize the importance of the heart and gut brains. It is necessary to support all three brains with specific nutritional supplements to achieve and maintain optimal performance on all levels.

Brain basics

- In order to get results when supporting the three brains, supplements need to contain meaningful amounts of their respective ingredients. One formula cannot provide the amounts required to have a therapeutic effect. Rather than taking five or six single-ingredient products and wondering if they are the most important, a "kit" called Daily Brain provides some of the most important nutritional supplements in an all-in-one packet to support the three brains. Daily Brain contains some of the most important three-brain supplements, such as phosphatidylserine, curcumin, omega-3 fatty acids, grapeseed extract, and probiotics.

- Essential fatty acids and phospholipids have been proven very beneficial for cognitive function and mental health in general, and additional supplementation provides extra insurance to protect the brain. Look for a combined omega-3 fatty acid/phospholipid formula such as Brilliant Mind, which contains omega-3 fatty acids, phosphatidylcholine, phosphatidylserine, L-alpha-glycerophosphorylcholine (alpha GPC), and green tea extract.

- A multivitamin and mineral supplement is also very important for optimal health of the three brains. It provides the nutrients often deficient in our North American diets. Look for a good quality ISURA-certified multivitamin and mineral supplement. A multivitamin will provide the necessary cofactors for the synthesis of neurotransmitters in the three brains, as well as antioxidant support.

- In addition to the brain basics mentioned above, specific brain disorders such as insomnia, depression, anxiety, and memory disorders may require additional supplemental support.

Brain basics for children

- In general, the same ideas associated with healthy eating in adults apply to children – lots of fresh fruit and veggies, complex carbohydrates, complete proteins, good fats, and, of course, drink lots of water.

- Most children do not get enough omega-3 fatty acids in their diets. Studies clearly show that essential fatty acids (EFAs) are crucial for optimal health and brain function in children. Because the brain is literally built from fatty acids, it makes sense that they play an integral role in brain development and function. Look for a combined form of omega-3 containing the two fatty acids, docosahexaenoic acid (DHA) and eicosapentaenoic acid (EPA), which are essential to brain function.

- Children and teens with attention deficit hyperactivity disorder (ADHD) and related learning difficulties are more likely to have low EFA levels and could benefit from supplementation. (Refer to Chapter 6 for more information on supplementation for learning problems in children and teens.)

- A children's multivitamin and mineral is very important to supply the basic nutrients missing from the diet that help support optimal brain function.

- Probiotics for children are crucial, not only for general health, but also to help prevent any mental, emotional, or learning problems related to imbalanced microbiota.

- For those who have the hyperactive/impulsive component to learning disorders, it is important to supplement the natural approach to treatment with a product that can help calm the central nervous system, such as gamma-aminobutyric acid (GABA), L-theanine, or lemon balm.

(Refer to Chapter 6 for more information on the importance of diet and nutrition in children.)

The "Not So Optimal" You – When You Start to Lose Your Identity

As discussed in Chapters 3 and 4, brain busters interfere with optimal performance of the three brains. Some people may experience temporary lapses in memory, brain fatigue, or mood changes, while others experience more severe symptoms related to learning disorders, anxiety, mood and depressive disorders, and debilitating memory conditions.

Stress

Stress affects the three brains in different ways and has a direct impact on the development of a variety of mental health disorders. Many studies show a correlation between stress and the development of cardiovascular disease, intestinal disorders, and mental health problems such as depression and other mood disorders, anxiety, insomnia, dementias including Alzheimer's disease, drug and alcohol abuse, and learning problems.

During times of increased demands or prolonged stress, many people begin to experience both physical and mental fatigue. They may be less able to maintain focus and attention, or experience sleep and anxiety problems. The following suggestions are ways to help reduce the impact of stress:

- Daily Brain, mentioned earlier, supports the three brains.

- Many supplements are available to help maintain mental and physical energy during times of increased stress. Look for a product such as Stress Less containing ashwagandha, rhodiola, *Panax ginseng*, green tea extract, and choline to help support the adrenal glands, the main stress-adaptive organs.

(Refer to Chapter 2 for more information and research on stress and the three brains.)

Sleep Disorders

According to Statistics Canada, one in seven Canadians has insomnia, which is characterized as the inability to fall asleep or to stay asleep, or to experience restorative sleep. According to the World Association of Sleep Medicine, sleep problems including insomnia, sleep apnea, restless legs syndrome, and sleep deprivation in general affect up to 45% of the world's population. The following suggestions are ways to help reduce the impact of sleep disorders:

- The gut and heart brains play important roles in the treatment of insomnia. New studies indicate that probiotics have beneficial effects on anxiety and reduce the stress hormone cortisol, a common cause of chronic insomnia. The heart brain is also involved in insomnia. It is well-known that overexcitement or worry can increase heart rate and elevate blood pressure, which also contribute to insomnia.

- Avoid stimulating foods such as coffee, chocolate, or sugars as they can increase the release of stress hormones, making insomnia worse. Instead, drink a soothing tea toward evening such as chamomile or linden flower. Rigorous exercise late in the day or early evening can also overstimulate the adrenal glands and make insomnia worse, so try to exercise in the morning.

- Stress support is important in the management of sleep problems. In fact, adrenal regulation is necessary in order to stop the vicious cycle of stress and insomnia. Stress Less, containing ashwagandha, rhodiola, *Panax ginseng*, green tea extract, and choline, provides support for the adrenal glands during times of stress. Remember that treating the adrenals takes time, so additional nutritional supplementation will most likely be necessary to treat more chronic insomnia.

- It is common for people with adrenal fatigue as a result of chronic stress to feel "tired but wired", so it is difficult to shut down the mind at night. Supplements such as kava kava, L-theanine, or GABA can help keep the system calm during the day, making it easier to fall asleep and stay asleep at night.

- Daily Brain, mentioned earlier, is not specifically for sleep, however it contains probiotics and other nutritional supplements that support the three brains.

- Look for a supplement such as Restful Sleep, containing passionflower, California poppy, skullcap powder, and linden flowers, to help with insomnia.

(Refer to Chapter 8 for more information on causes and treatment options for insomnia and other sleep disorders.)

Inflammation

Inflammation is a protective reaction that aids in the repair and regeneration of damaged cells. If it continues for too long, however, inflammation does more harm than good, contributing to depression and other mood disorders, as well as dementias, cardiovascular disease, intestinal disorders, and joint problems. Inflammation affects all three brains. Canadian researchers have found that a protein known to be a marker of inflammation is up to one-third higher in the brains of depressed patients compared to healthy ones. In addition, those with the most severe forms of depression have the most inflammation.

Chronic inflammation causes an imbalance between the overproduction of free radicals and the ability of antioxidants to protect the cells. Free radicals damage cells by reacting with proteins and cell membrane fatty acids, and can impair their function permanently. The most important step in preventing free radical damage is to prevent or treat inflammation. The following suggestions are ways to help reduce and prevent inflammation:

- Look for an anti-inflammatory/cognition formula such as Brain Defence, containing bacopa, ashwagandha, curcumin, chamomile, and boswellia.

- Look for an ISURA-certified omega-3 fatty acid supplement containing eicosapentaenoic acid (EPA) and docosahexaenoic acid (DHA). (Refer to Chapter 5 for more information on omega-3 fatty acids.) Note: Omega-3 fatty acids may increase the effects of blood thinning medications such as aspirin or warfarin.

(Refer to Chapter 2 for more for more information on stress and Chapter 3 for more information on inflammation.)

Mood Disorders

Mood disorders affect about 15% of the population in Canada, with depression and anxiety being the most common. Imbalance in the neurotransmitters (chemical messengers) in the brains that are involved in anxiety and mood disorders can be caused by various factors seldom addressed in Western medicine. These include stress and other factors such as inflammation, blood sugar problems, allergies, heavy metals, high-sugar diet, faulty gut-brain axis, and heart abnormalities. These factors are seldom addressed in Western medicine.

Anxiety and depression

- Stress is often a causative factor in mood disorders, and studies have shown that phosphatidylserine (PS) can offset the body's response to physical stress by decreasing the level of stress hormones. Probiotics are also being explored in the treatment of depressive disorders. In addition, depression and anxiety appear to be linked to lower levels of omega-3 fatty acids. Look for an all-in-one brain kit such as Daily Brain that contains probiotics, omega-3 fatty acids, and PS, as well as other important supplements for three-brain health.

- For those with mood disorders who experience chronic stress, consider trying an all-in-one formulation such as Look for Stress Less, which contains ashwagandha, rhodiola, *Panax ginseng*, green tea extract, and choline.

- Studies have shown that inositol, saffron, and 5-HTP have proven beneficial in the treatment of mood disorders and depressive disorders. Look for a formula such as Cloud Nine that contains inositol, saffron, 5-HTP, and vitamin B-6.

- New research is finding that inflammation is a significant contributing factor in depression. Look for a formula such as Brain Defence, which contains bacopa, ashwagandha, curcumin, chamomile, and boswellia to prevent or help with the inflammation related to depression.

Mood swings

- Mood swings are commonly caused by dramatic changes in blood sugar levels. People love their carbohydrates, especially the refined variety, and as a result blood sugar imbalance is very common in our society. Chromium supplementation has been shown to alleviate hypoglycemic symptoms.

- Soluble dietary fibre plays an important role in stabilizing blood sugar levels. PGX® (PolyGlycopleX) is a completely new and unique fibre matrix. The effectiveness of any fibre for reducing appetite, blood sugar, and cholesterol is based on the amount of water the fibre is able to absorb. The health benefits linked to soluble dietary fibre – including stabilizing blood sugar levels – are significantly magnified with PGX. For more information on the benefits of PGX please refer to www.pgx.com.

(Refer to Chapter 7 for more information on mood disorders such as depression, anxiety, and mood swings.)

Memory Loss

Age-related memory loss

Everyone experiences forgetfulness at one time or another, like misplacing keys, blanking on someone's name, or forgetting a phone number or the title of a movie you recently saw. A younger person may not pay much attention to these lapses, but as we grow older, sometimes we worry about what they mean. Age-related memory changes are not the same thing as dementia.

While it is true that certain brain changes are inevitable when it comes to aging, major memory problems are not one of them and are preventable in most cases. New research now indicates that memory loss is not simply due to the head brain, but also has gut brain and heart brain involvement. The following suggestions are ways to help with age-related memory loss:

- Research has shown that PS can slow, halt, or reverse the decline of memory and mental function due to aging. There is increasing evidence that supplementation with PS can improve mood, learning, and concentration, as well as specific brain disorders including seasonal affective disorder (SAD), depression, ADHD, and Alzheimer's. PS also helps young, healthy people cope with anxiety, neuroticism, and stress. (Refer to Chapters 3 and 9 for more information.)

- Diet and lifestyle factors, as well as specific nutritional support for the three brains, supply the necessary nutrients and cofactors to keep the brains healthy throughout the lifespan. Look for an all-in-one kit such as Daily Brain containing some of the most important three-brain supplements, such as phosphatidylserine, curcumin, omega-3 fatty acids, grapeseed extract, and probiotics.

- For those people in midlife who are starting to experience age-related memory problems, extra supplement support in addition to Daily Brain provides added insurance and helps prevent further decline. Look for a formula such as Brilliant Mind, which contains phosphatidylserine, phosphatidylcholine, omega-3 fatty acids, L-alpha-glycerophosphorylcholine, and green tea extract.

- For those experiencing changes in memory due to chronic stress, Stress Less contains ashwagandha, rhodiola, *Panax ginseng*, green tea extract, and choline. (Refer to Chapter 2 for more information on stress and its effects on the three brains.)

- Addressing the inflammation in the body can not only help prevent mental health and memory disorders, but also other conditions associated with inflammation such as cardiovascular disease, arthritis, and gut disorders, to name a few. Look for a supplement such as Brain Defence, which contains bacopa, ashwagandha, curcumin, chamomile, and boswellia to prevent and treat inflammation and to help support cognition and memory.

Dementia-related memory problems

Alzheimer's is the most common type of dementia. "Dementia" is an umbrella term describing a variety of diseases and conditions that develop when nerve cells in the brain (called neurons) die or no longer function normally. The death or malfunction of neurons causes changes in memory, behaviour, and the ability to think clearly, and in some cases results in the complete loss of identity.

Several different factors involving the three brains can contribute to the development of dementias, including stress hormones, gut microbiota imbalances, gluten intolerance and other allergies, pesticides and heavy metal toxicity, thyroid disorders, blood sugar disorders, cardiovascular disease, inflammation, and free radical damage. Here again you can see the involvement of the heart, gut, and head brains in the development of dementias. The following suggestions are ways to help with dementia-related memory problems:

- Follow the nutritional support recommendations mentioned in the previous section.

- Additional antioxidant and cognitive support may be necessary for those experiencing longer term or more advanced memory loss such as dementia. Phospholipids such as phosphatidylserine and antioxidants like N-acetyl-L-cysteine (NAC) and lipoic acid have proven very beneficial in preventing and treating memory loss. Look for a product such as Brain & Memory Boost that combines acetyl-L-carnitine, NAC, alpha-lipoic acid, *ginkgo biloba,* phosphatidylserine, vinpocetine, and huperzia serrata extract.

(Refer to Chapter 9 for more detailed information and research on some of the possible causes, as well as lab tests and dietary and nutritional suggestions, for memory loss and dementias. Refer to Chapter 5 for more information on dietary recommendations and the importance of water.)

The more information you have about a specific health problem, the more you will understand what can be done to improve your mental, emotional, and physical well-being. I invite you to review the concept of the three brains in Chapter 1 and throughout this book and consider how the integration and support of these three information centres can lead to improved overall health. Use Three Brains; How the Heart, Brain, and Gut Influence Mental Health and Identity as a guide to learn as much as possible to prevent and support symptoms of many common mental health disorders. The information provided can help you attain and maintain optimal three-brain health.